Gianmaria Benedetti

The Autism Bubble

We need to abandon the wrong concept of autism
and to change the approach to the difficulties
of children's psychic development.

Editorial note: this book is published in Italian and English, both as a paper and e-book. It includes some partially modified texts written separately and at different times for my websites. I apologize for the inevitable repetitions.
The cover is by Sara Francesconi.

To my wife

Index

INTRODUCTION

This book stems from the need to denounce a situation becoming more and more akin to a health emergency which is not mentioned in the public domain. An increasing number of little children and their families, are being plunged into a tunnel of questionable and unproven tests and therapies that disrupt their lives. All this is happening because of the psychosis of autism spreading everywhere, in health care and in schools, kindergartens and wherever children are concerned, not to mention newspapers, TV and the web spreading alarmism and untruths without limits. The development of this situation now threatens the health of children and families with small children. It has been caused by the growth of what now appears to be a veritable speculative bubble and perhaps a lobby of conflicting interests about an entity, autism, whose existence was never really demonstrated.

There have been many international reports denouncing the need to completely change the approach in the field of children's developmental difficulties, which this 'autism bubble' has virtually incorporated all together without distinction. But everything is silent in the public domain, or at least criticisms, doubts and uncertainties remain confined to restricted spaces without reaching the media and the attention of public opinion. At the institutional level further transformations and reorganizations of health care are menacingly promoted to precipitate this situation. The issue of autism has therefore become a matter of general, national and international health interest which threatens the health of children and families and needs to be deepened and clarified. I believe that it is no longer possible to remain silent or simply to express criticisms of this increasingly serious situation in our private or in closed sector of scientific and professional associations. The intent of this book is to draw attention explicitly to these aspects by openly addressing these important issues. Children must be released from these diagnostic bubbles in which they are locked up due to seriously flawed health practices that risk profoundly disrupting their development. In these bubbles children become invisible to parents, doctors, teachers, who no longer see the child as a person in his or her entirety and characteristics. They only see automata that "do not indicate", "do not respond" and "do not greet on demand" and must be trained like robots or circus animals. Like in the days of Hamelin's Pied Piper, we risk losing our children because we are not aware of what is really happening.

Chapter 1

What's this about?

The current situation is this: in this period many parents with young children are living the dramatic experience of seeing their child thrown, for often trivial reasons, into the autism test tunnel. The term 'tunnel' is used by many parents who have had this experience. So if their 18 month old child doesn't speak yet, if he or she is a little behind his or her developmental peers, if he or she doesn't cooperate enough with a visit to the paediatrician, the question arises "could he or she be autistic". Anxiety and alarm often begins to spread even before the child turns one year old: more and more anxious mothers and fathers fear they recognize symptoms of autism in children just a few months old; they panic and fill their relationship with the child with worries and begin to bombard him with tests and trials with the risk of actually disturbing the child's evolution.

It may be the parents themselves who resort to the paediatrician for the doubts fuelled by reading the internet pages that list the symptoms and signs of autism, or the paediatrician himself at the scheduled visit of 18 months that finds some 'suspicious' aspect in the child, 'a wake-up call', it is said, and here the child is sent to a specialist or directly to an autism centre. It's as if every child with the first cough is suspected of having tuberculosis, pneumonia and whatever else and is hospitalized for invasive and disturbing tests. In reality, a real psychosis has been created among parents, pediatricians, health and school workers, not to mention relatives, friends and neighbors, who see symptoms of autism in a great many children and thus push an increasing number of families to access diagnostic services for autism, which have sprung up in recent years like mushrooms both in the public and private sectors.

So the family begins its specialist procedure. The first specialist consulted is usually a child psychiatrist, who sees the child usually for quite a short time, confirms possible suspicions and almost inevitably directs for further examination to the centres for the specific diagnosis of autism. On the other hand, the guidelines say so. Here, the child and the parents are interviewed and observed to collect data on the child's behavior at home and during the visit, on his or her abilities, etc. The child is often evaluated, especially if the Centre is quite big and famous, by different operators (psychomotricist, speech therapist, pedagogist, behavioral analyst, etc.) in more or less long times (many months in the public, obviously clogged by the plethora of cases, less in the private one). The data collected are included in the charts provided by the most common behavioral tests (ADOS, ADI, CHAT, etc.) with the scores measuring the performance of the children, their abilities and their behaviors, attributed by the testers on the basis of the observations during the sessions or the answers of the parents, and the sum of these scores establishes a rating according to which the child is put in different boxes. And finally it is an algorithm, it is said, perhaps to make the atmosphere aseptic, which evaluates the data collected and the scores and establishes the diagnosis of all the children. A more or less long report is then drawn up and given to the family with all the data collected, tables, scores, explanations and instructions for use, and finally the algebraic diagnosis, so to speak, with numerical references to the classifications in vogue.

The family returns at this point to the child psychiatrist who had started the procedure and the latter, quickly scrolling through the sheets with the scores and calculations made, promulgates the fateful diagnosis. It is usually a diagnosis without appeal. Whether the response is of mild, medium or severe autistic spectrum, or in rare cases of borderline position, i.e. risk of falling within the spectrum, it is communicated that without a shadow of a doubt or margin of error the child is suffering from an Autistic Spectrum Disorder, which is certainly genetic in nature, which is incurable, but for which it is necessary to make early and massive educational interventions that can reduce his disabilities and make him learn skills, relationality, communication, which otherwise he would never learn.

And so it begins the process, immediately if you resort to the private sector, after months or years if you stay in public. It is practically the same for everyone - so much so that it is the same Disorder! - regardless of the level of gravity, often recommended even to children miraculously "out of the spectrum". The result is sessions of psychomotricity and speech therapy and behavioral therapy, a triad that smells of holiness.[1] These 'therapies' take up many hours a week, sometimes in different and distant places, and often disrupt family life and make it difficult to attend nursery or kindergarten.

Of these children, some still improve and continue their development - there is no way to know whether as a result of the interventions or simply the maturation of the child; some remain unchanged and some get worse and face further crises. The statistics on the development of cases are very scarce and unreliable, especially if they are produced by centers and schools that promote themselves.

It was common experience, in unsuspected times, in the first decades after the appearance of the autistic syndrome, that a part of autistic children healed or improved, independently of treatment or not, and some became capable of autonomous and independent living, a part maintained mild or medium difficulties and a part remained at the level of severe mental handicap.

It is worthwhile to go through the historical evolution of this issue a little bit.

---

[1]This description refers to Italian situation, the reader will compare it with what happens elsewhere.

Chapter 2

Recent Historical Excursus

The following are some ideas that reflect a change in my way of considering the field of phenomena hitherto collected under the name of autism, which I have been dealing with since the beginning of my working experience.

I remember that it was 1973 when I was a first-year resident in the child neuro-psychiatry ward in Careggi, Florence University (Italy), and I met the first child with this diagnosis: ten years of age, without language, without communication and symbolic learning, his behavior revealed a certain intelligence that he used to get what he needed and to keep under his control what was happening immediately around him. I met and then worked professionally for a long time with other 'autistic' boys and girls and families with children with autism within them, trying to help the development of those children and families.

The world of psychiatry faced great changes in those years all over the world. In Italy these led to health care reform and the closure of asylums, in 1978, with the so-called Basaglia law (the name of the psychiatrist who was the main promoter of the change), as well as the closure of special schools and the inclusion of children with disabilities in normal schools, together with all other children. Others methodological and taxonomic changes arrived in Italy a decade later, under the banner of a methodology more attentive to observable phenomena and less to pathogenetic hypotheses. One of these changes, for child psychiatry, was the diagnostic voice of 'pervasive developmental disorders', which arrived in the early 1980s together with DSM 3 (the American classification, previously little followed in Europe), which collected in one diagnostic category the classic autistic syndrome plus some similar clinical pictures but with different characteristics, badly framed, "not otherwise classifiable".

I was impressed by this conceptualization because it emphasized 'development' instead of 'disease' ('psychosis'): it was globally disturbed in those cases, while other children were disturbed in more limited areas of the person, language, learning, etc.. The fact of considering things from the point of view of 'development', instead of 'disease' - often considered from the perspective of adult diseases, as has long been the case in the childhood field, see 'schizophrenia', 'psychosis', etc. - seemed to me that could help us to see more clearly, in a situation that continued to elude any attempt at real understanding.

Initially, even the concept of a 'spectrum' - in the physical sense, like the spectrum of colors that follow one another in the rainbow and in the refraction of a ray of white light through a glass prism - seemed useful to bring together disparate phenomena that seem to have something in common, like a continuum.

The field of observation was that of psychic development and the alterations it could undergo, giving rise to similar and different syndromes at the same time. I had tried myself with other colleagues to account for such similarities and differences, starting from the investigation in psychoanalytic therapy of children with autism about so called autistic mental state and other mental states observable in session, according to the D.Meltzer's and Tavistock Clinic model[2]. The detractors of psychoanalysis generally have no idea about that, as they usually consider only the classic Freudian approaches of the first decades of the 20th century.

But the individual psychotherapies of children with autism were less and less applicable, both because of the strain of age (for me) and because of the retreating phase of psychoanalysis under 'military occupation' by cognitive-behavioral troops. I was also increasingly convinced by focalizing on the whole environment, which was already present in the idea of creating a total therapeutic environment at home, school, therapy centers - in the setting up of the center which I had been working on for some years - and which I had then tried to set up in the peripheral work, on the 'territory', as it was said and perhaps still is said, at the Health Agency (ASL) of Florence.

From the 1990's onwards also in Italy the field of autism and child development was increasingly invaded by

---

[2] Meltzer, D., et al. (1975). *Explorations in Autism: A Psycho-Analytical Study*, Karnac Books Ltd.

neopositivist diagnostic and therapeutic methods, based on tables and measurements made with tests and lists of symptoms, with a mechanical-biological vision that excluded from its perspective the person, his or her life experiences and relationships. The origin was from the American world, especially, but also behaviorist England gave its contribution, for example with the ADOS test of M. Rutter and C., which spread like the weed, until it became the diagnostic method par excellence in the diagnosis of autism. It has to be said, however, in defense of the first extenders, that its application has been seriously misrepresented, going beyond their intentions, to become almost an omnipotent magic tool given into the hands of operators who otherwise lacked a wider clinical experience: a dangerous weapon in the hands of unaware and often fanatical people.

These new approaches seemed to make 'tabula rasa' of any previous experience. A mechanical and dogmatic vision of development, of the characteristics of the person and his psychological abilities was imposed everywhere. It happened almost all over the world, also thanks to lobbies that in Italy went as far as parliament to induce specific laws for autism, elsewhere as far as the UN and the World Health Organization. The relationship with patients and families was also transformed into something mechanical and aseptic, lacking the ability to deal with the difficult psychological implications of a diagnosis of autism.

The effect was to once again transform the developmental-centered viewpoint into a disease-centered viewpoint. The claim was and is to dogmatically establish, without the necessary scientific evidence, the neurobiological nature of autism and the 'autistic spectrum' as a behavioral syndrome caused by specific biological abnormalities of a genetic nature. As a mantra it is repeated everywhere that genetic and biochemical research is on the verge of discovering or being increasingly close to definitively revealing the causes of autism. Which hasn't happened so far, as it seems.

So a new specter is haunting Europe and the world, the 'Autistic Spectrum' - increasingly extended to include almost every child with difficulties of neuropsychic development. This is causing an epidemic increase in the number of cases diagnosed: up to 1 in every 38 children, in the most recent statistical claims! The idea of a neurobiological abnormality underlying the characteristics and disorders of the conditions collected in the 'spectrum' determines the belief in pre-existing diseases before of the onset of symptoms and which had to be sought from the first doubts, or even before they occurred, extending screening to 'asymptomatic cases' and also to adults possible healthy carriers or 'below threshold' cases, according to a well-known local School.

Every child with minimal delays and difficulties - indeed every child, even healthy ones - can thus be autistic and must be tested. At the same time, sensing business opportunity, centers and organizations are multiplying on the market that propagate 'timely diagnosis and immediate treatment', of a strictly cognitive-behavioral nature, obviously, at least while waiting for the miracle drug that everyone is waiting for. Even if "the Disorder" is called "incurable", the idea promoted is that the earlier the diagnosis and intervention, the more extensive the recovery of capacity and the lesser the disability.

Almost as in the plague or cholera epidemics of past centuries, panic is spreading. At the same time, sellers of all kinds of miracle remedies for autism are multiplying, and centers offering fashionable therapies. Many unfortunate families go everywhere and do everything, falling into dangerous traps and endless tunnels, often making their situation worse.

This seems to me to be the situation in recent years. My activity had gradually turned in my field to counter this abnormal extension of diagnosis of autism, in the new name of Autistic Spectrum which devastated the lives of the families I met. I considered, like other colleagues of mine, that these were serious diagnostic errors, the result of methodological errors and specialist training influenced by bad teachers.

Then I happened to read Dr. Lynn Waterhouse's book, which will be discussed in the next chapter, and something struck me, so to speak, precipitating a mental reaction whose components had been present for a long time, there was just something missing to connect them. If this new idea turns out to be full of potential developments or disappears without a trace it will be seen in time. The result, perhaps the beginning of a possible change, you can read about it on the following pages.

Chapter 3

Brief historical overview of the term 'autism' and its applications

The term 'autism' (from the Greek autòs, meaning itself, with various nuances) was coined at the beginning of the 20th century by the director of the Zurich asylum, psychiatrist Eugen Bleuler, who also coined the term 'schizophrenia'. He described with that term the behavior/symptom of many schizophrenic patients in his hospital, who closed in on themselves and paid little or no attention to the world around them. Since they had often been in asylums for several years, and knowing what asylums were like, perhaps their 'symptom' was not so strange, but psychiatry mostly did not (does not...) take the environment into account.

Also in Switzerland, the Geneva psychologist J Piaget used the term 'autistic' in the 1930s, but in another context, to describe what he considered a transitory phase of the development of thought and language in children, in the development period he called 'childish egocentricity'. In this case 'autistic' was used in the sense of 'addressed to himself and not yet to others'.

Then Leo Kanner, an Austrian child psychiatrist who emigrated to America after the First World War, used the term 'autistic' applying it to children. In the early 1940s he coined the formula 'early childhood autism' to give a diagnostic label to a group of children who attracted his attention. Although very different from each other, they had in common a marked detachment and closure from the environment and particular behaviors. Since then, the term 'autism' has become established in medical use and diagnosis. Kanner himself, faced with the spread of his diagnosis, warned against the risk of turning it into a cauldron to contain the most diverse things.[3]

More or less at the same time another Austrian doctor, Dr Hans Asperger had used the term 'autistic' for children whom he called 'autistic psychopaths' - and perhaps handed some of them over to the Nazis after the annexation of Austria to the Third Reich, for the Nazi program of elimination of the mentally ill (as Herwig Czech writes in a recent well-documented article [4]). Before that, in 1926, a Russian doctor, named Grunya Sukhareva, had called a group of similar children 'schizoid psychopaths'. In those years, Russia was being traversed by groups of children abandoned to themselves, torn and hungry, living on gimmicks, which only recently has been mentioned again (L.

---

[3] Kanner, *Child Psychiatry, 1957,* C C Thomas Publisher

[4] Herwig Czech, *Hans Asperger, National Socialism, and "race hygiene" in Nazi-era Vienna, Molecular Autism,* 2018-
https://molecularautism.biomedcentral.com/articles/10.1186/s13229-018-0208-6

Mecacci[5]). In the same years the psychoanalyst Melanie Klein described what in retrospect was considered the first example of psychoanalytic treatment of an autistic child. However, she spoke of 'schizophrenia', albeit with reservations. We'll go back to it in the Appendices. In the following years a German doctor, who came out of Germany to escape Nazism, named Lula Wolff, in Scotland, took care of children whom she described as 'schizoids' and recognized as similar to Sukhareva and Asperger's cases.

In all these cases, most of them hospitalized in psychiatric wards and children's institutions, no mention was made of the environmental conditions, except, in passing, in M. Klein's report.

'Autistic' and 'schizoid' were therefore adjectives used in an equivalent way, for a period of time, until the concept of 'autistic spectrum' encompassed all these terms. Thus the children in question were finally brought together into one label, differentiating them only on a scale of gravity. The 'cauldron' feared and preconceived by Kanner had come true.

In all these situations it was always argued that the causes were 'inborn', 'genetic', and that environmental situations and families should not be blamed. These, as is well known, were initially called into question by Kanner and, in his wake, by psychiatrists and psychoanalysts such as Bruno Bettelheim, Margaret Mahler, Frances Tustin and others. Indeed, it was pontificated that "Scientific Research" had shown that the environmental and family situation had nothing to do with it.

---

[5]Mecacci,L.*Besprizornye*, Adelphi Edizioni, 2019

Obviously, it was not a question of 'faults', but of possible environmental causes linked to the life experiences of the various families, that is, to possible psycho-social factors. These, in modern bio-psycho-social psychiatry, are widely recognized concausal factors for most psychological and psychiatric difficulties.

Indeed, from the 1970s onwards, because of this myth or specter of 'parental guilt', it became taboo to deal with the environmental conditions in which children considered 'autistic' grew up. Any hypothesis of environmental influence on their psychic development was declared unreliable and 'unscientific'. It was officially declared that autism and the autistic spectrum are 'neurodevelopmental disorders' due to causes that are certainly genetic. And this is the official position of 'science' today. But of this, as it was said, there is not the slightest proof, it is only the belief of the 'authorities' in the matter: a truth supported only by 'ipse dixit', the basic criterion of medieval Scholasticism, which is certainly not the maximum of the scientific method.

Only recently, due to the failure of genetics to identify precise causes at the level of specific genes, a possible environmental component is being called into question here and there. This would have a triggering effect on the manifestation of the syndrome, and one suddenly realizes that there is a lack of studies on the subject. Among other things, in a timid resumption of scientific research on environmental aspects, recent studies are showing that environmental experiences, in particular abuse and neglect, have a visible effect on the anatomical growth and functioning of certain areas of the brain. (C Zeanah[6]). This recent research seems to show that even in the brain 'function creates structure', as an old medical adage used to say.

A mention should be made of so-called 'institutional autism'; this term came into vogue in the 1990s, in studies and reports of adopted children from orphanages in Eastern Europe in the last decade of the last century. It was noted that several of these children had signs and symptoms that overlapped with those of autistic children. If the stay in the institution was not too long and if the adoption experience was positive, these children lost autistic characteristics quite quickly and resumed their development (See Appendix 3).

Someone may remember that similar observations were made after World War II by psychoanalysts such as René Spitz, Anna Freud and others who had taken care of English children during the war. On the other hand, it is not out of place the observation that still in the 70s and 80s in Italy in children's institutions, there were many cases of autism, among others in children and young people with trisomy 21, while now children with this genetic syndrome show almost no more symptoms of autism. It would seem a clear sign, almost for a social experiment, of the importance of environmental conditions for normal and pathological psychological development.

---

[6]Zeanah C. H, Sonuga-Barke E.J.S. *Editorial: The effects of early trauma and deprivation on human development – from measuring cumulative risk to characterizing specific mechanisms,* J Child Psychol Psychiatry. 2016 Oct;57(10):1099-102. doi: 10.1111/jcpp.12642.

Chapter 4

About the neurobiological theories of autism.

Many things are said about autism, about its manifestations, about its diagnostic criteria (which vary every
given time inducing an accordion effect on the number of
cases included), about its causes, (defined almost by law as
neurobiological), about its therapies (which in Italy, by law
of the Parliament, must be 'educational-behavioral'); about
its prognosis (that is said as obviously negative "if not
cured in time"), and so on. But it is not said, or is it very
difficult to say, what it is: a disease, a way of being, a type
of personality? As for other 'mental illnesses', as they were
once called with less hypocrisy, the term 'disorder' has been
coined, a word that perhaps expresses the fact that these
'things' disturb public order and peace. In fact, the definitions of autism found on both official and popular sites
show the difficulties of dealing with this concept.

A current official version of autism reads "Autism is
a behavioral syndrome caused by a biologically determined
developmental disorder, beginning in the first three years

of life." [7] In an Italian pediatric popular site it is written: "Autism is a set of alterations in brain development, variable from one subject to another, which involve an impairment of social skills and language, as well as various behavioral disorders" [8].

The American Centers for Disease Control and Prevention states: "Autistic Spectrum Disorder (DSA) is a developmental disability that can cause significant social, communication and behavioral challenges" [9]. A popular Australian website states: "Autistic Spectrum Disorder (DSA) is a brain-based developmental condition. Children with DSA have communication difficulties, narrow interests and repetitive behavior" [10].

Behavioral syndrome, developmental disability, developmental condition, set of alterations in brain development: the terms are as vague and uncertain in the definition of the object as rigidly fixed in its causality, "biologically determined", "brain-based". etc. They say that this object is a biological, cerebral, genetic one, etc., but we cannot see it in any way and we do not know exactly what it is.

Leo Kanner in his Handbook of Child Psychiatry, third edition, 1957, wrote: "In 1943 I described eleven cas-

---

[7] Società Italiana Neuropsichiatria Infanzia Adolescenza, *Linee guida per l'autismo, 2011,* Erikson Ed

[8] Calia V., *autismo e disturbi dello spettro autistico*. Un pediatra per amico , 4/11/'19 https://www.uppa.it/medicina/malattie-e-disturbi/autismo-disturbi-dello-spettro-autistico/

[9] Centers for Disease Control and Prevention, *What is ASD,* https://www.cdc.gov/ncbddd/autism/facts.html/

[10] Raisingchildren.net.au, *ASD: overview*, https://raisingchildren.net.au/autism/learning-about-asd/about-asd/asd-overview/

es of children who tended to lock themselves up from their first year of life. I suggested the term early childhood autism for this condition." The picture was inserted in the chapter of childhood schizophrenia, the general causes of which were obscure. Among other things, on page 725 of the Italian edition it is written, "from a purely statistical point of view, the correlation of schizophrenia with parental attitudes is much closer and higher than with other factors (inheritance, somatic substrate, metabolic disorders)". A few lines below he adds "...life experiences had confused these children, made interpersonal relationships impossible and induced them to shut themselves in...". This is to recall what Kanner wrote.

Since Kanner's time, not much has changed in the knowledge of the causes and nature of the condition he described. What has changed is the approach of psychiatry which, since the middle of the last century, has made a decisive choice of field between psychology and medicine, and has tried and is trying to find its place as a medical specialty. For this reason, it has embraced the external characteristics of Evidence Based Medicine and tried to reduce its object, that is, 'disturbed' human behavior, to such dimensions that it can be inserted in the medical-biological box. A bit like Cinderella's sisters who had to cut off pieces of their feet to try to slip them into their glass slippers. So psychiatry has renounced so many parts of its object that it has often been reduced to a parody of medicine, imitating and ape-mimicking its vices, languages and manias, no longer taking care of people and their worries but only of their dysfunctional brains.

In reality the terms 'condition', 'disability', 'syndrome', 'set of alterations' express the difficulty of defining the concept of autism. What is this thing? Is it a disease? If we look for the explanation of other medical words and diagnosis, for example multiple sclerosis, hemochromatosis, diabetes, muscular dystrophy, etc., we invariably find that they are 'diseases' with particular characteristics, etiopathogenesis and causes. But with autism? Perhaps it is easier to consider it a symptom: closure in oneself. And the term was born from this and is useful to describe a behavior. Just as 'paralysis' indicates a difficulty of movement, or 'syncope' and 'coma' indicate transient or continuous loss of consciousness, 'autism' etymologically means closure in oneself. The autism symptom then, far from finding its cause, magically transformed, thanks to Kanner at first, into an entity that should explain the symptoms tautologically: from 'autistic symptom' to 'early childhood autism', to 'Pervasive Disorder' to 'Autistic Spectrum' in subsequent editions of the DSM. Almost an illusionistic game. At this point, having obtained the qualification of Disorder, everyone's attention focused on the definition of diagnostic criteria, classification categories and diagnostic methods and tools. We moved from the search for what it was to the description of its attributes, qualities, etc., without any longer dealing with the evidence of its existence. How to move from the subject if angels, demons, witches and goblins exist, to their detailed description and classification. All this without any 'evidence' of proof of the existence of the organic, cerebral, etc. causes of these disorders.

We refer to the next chapter the discussion of the failure of neurobiological research on autism, documented by Lynn Waterhouse in her landmark book.

The above definitions and statements about the nature of autism and its causes claim to be based on scientific data, but they are not. They are therefore revealed as aspects of a real propaganda and advertising action, which is repeated everywhere to the point of exhaustion, hoping that they end up passing as acquired knowledge.

On the website of the American Psychiatric Association, Childhood and Adolescence Sector, page on Autistic Spectrum Disorders, it reads: "What is autism?" The text states that autism spectrum disorders "are neurological disorders, i.e. they affect the functioning of the brain...". This sentence already has a disconcerting effect: neurological diseases (Epilepsy, Parkinson's disease, ALS, multiple sclerosis, and many others) have clear symptoms and objective signs on neurological examination, and several medical examinations show pathological brain abnormalities. Even there, much remains to be known about causes and therapies and diagnostic criteria vary over time according to interests perhaps not only scientific. But autism has no specific neurological symptoms and 'evidence' such as the diseases mentioned above, nor even less tests that document significant brain abnormalities. But autism has no specific neurological symptoms, such as the diseases mentioned above, nor, even less, tests and 'evidence' that document significant brain abnormalities. It only has behavioral symptoms: if any-thing, we should speak of a psychiatric disorder, not 'neurological'..., since it shares these characteristics with psychiatric disorders.

That then a part of psychiatry claims that mental disorders are only brain disorders is something else, but at least we would have clarified a linguistic sophistry. Psychiatry in these decades has made a real revolution in terms and expressions, and assembled a new construction of words, which have replaced those in force until a few decades ago. Whether the change in words is matched by a change in the underlying reality is another matter.

Continuing reading the text, they then talk about symptoms, diagnoses, treatments, advice to parents and, of course, causes. And here we read: "The exact causes of autism spectrum disorders are not clear. *Probably* (emphasis added) many factors contribute to autism, including the genes with which a child is born and possible environmental factors...". It specifies then: "research has shown that (autism) is not caused by bad parenting nor by vaccines...".

The text here resembles more of a political or advertising message (or a stereotypical jargon towards some deified lobby) than scientific information. These gentlemen talk about 'neurological disorders' (i.e., as in the various neurological diseases, 'disorders' resulting from alterations of the brain and its nerve cells) but then they say that the causes are not clear. It is true that there are many diseases, neurological and others, whose causes are unknown, but as I was saying, the anatomical and histological and instrumental findings that establish that the nervous system is involved are known. When you then say 'probably', you can say everything and the opposite of everything and it is clear that the statement cannot have safety value, like the one with which it is said that they are neurological disorders.

In the midst of this sea of probability, the obviously 'political' addition on bad parenting, where it is said that research has shown that parental attitudes and behavior are not involved, is the icing on the cake. Among other things, the expression is confusing, perhaps intentionally: it confuses the possibility of negative, traumatic environmental experiences with a moralistic judgment of parents, with the effect of reinforcing the taboo on research on relational and educational environmental factors, as we describe in another chapter. There is in fact no specific evidence: if, as they say, the factors at stake are '*probably*' different, how can we safely exclude some of them? What can be said is that so far there is no definite evidence of anything, neither genetic nor immune or toxic factors, nor 'human', relational environmental factors: but neither can we exclude them, given that genetic and toxic and immune mechanisms are at stake in many known diseases and similarly well known human and social environmental factors are at stake. It is more honest in my opinion to say that for the moment we do not have sufficient knowledge to express ourselves.

The same applies to possible remedies and therapies. As we are not certain about the causes and factors involved, interventions can only be symptomatic, dictated by situations, and if possible based on common sense. Not having a clear definition and demarcation of the limits of a situation, we cannot have a specific object on which to evaluate treatments and prognosis.

Out of curiosity it may be useful to examine a definition and a series of current questions and answers in Italy at a popular level on Autism and autism spectrum disorders, from the point of view of the Autism System. For this we refer to Appendix 5.

Chapter 5

Rethinking autism

A book published in America in 2013 by Dr Lynn Waterhouse, "Rethinking Autism" [11], has raised an underlying critical wave that has affected the entire cathedral built around autism. The book extensively examines a quantity of data and research results of the last twenty years, on the causes, symptoms, evolution and treatment of autism to conclude that so many efforts and so much funding have practically failed to find a cause and a cure. She even states that autism does not exist as a single disorder, but only autistic symptoms exist which, like fever, are not a disease in themselves, but the result of different causes. The book also talks about current therapies as being con-

---

[11]Waterhouse L., *Rethinking-Autism* Academic Press, 2012 - The author is an authoritative person in the field: the editorial info's tells us that she was "Director of Child Behavior Study at The College of New Jersey for 31 years" and is currently "Professor in Global Graduate Programs at the College NIMH, NICHD". We are also informed that she worked with Dr. Lorna Wing at the DSM-III-R to establish diagnostic criteria for autism.

ducted blindly, since they are not based on a knowledge of possible brain abnormalities in individual cases.

The author identifies among the causes of errors that have led to this failure some of the cornerstones of the theory of autism today dominant, such as the concept of the Autistic Spectrum itself and then that of 'comorbidity' that has infested psychiatry in recent years, and invites the scientific community to get rid of these errors that prevent the progress in knowledge. The same DSM5, the bible of American psychiatry that has been imposed on the world and its classification of Autistic Spectrum Disorders, are according to Waterhouse to be discarded if one wants to make progress in research.

In my opinion, the book represents an epitaph, if not on the whole current psychiatry and its methods, on at least two decades of scientific research on autism and on the theories that led it to a 'neurobiological disorder' as well as on the therapeutic methods that have spread like wildfire in the world in recent years. The conclusion of the book is precisely that so much effort and so much money have been useless, have not led to any real increase in knowledge about the phenomenon of autism, but rather the dominant conceptions have even blocked possible developments towards new knowledge.

The book identifies the main cause of this failure in the evident or hidden purpose that has moved the researchers in recent years, that is to find a unifying (biological) theory in the complexity and heterogeneity of autism cases and that would account for their common etiopathogenesis. The author states that none of the various theories advanced in these years, both biochemical, physiopathological, psychological and environmental, have proved reliable. On the basis of all the data, therefore, it must be concluded, says Waterhouse, that a specific pathology responsible for autism does not exist and there is not even an 'autism' in itself, nor a spectrum of related disorders. There are autistic symptoms variously combined and sometimes connected with known brain anomalies (for which we used to speak of secondary autism) or vice versa without obvious brain anomalies (for which we spoke of primary autism).

The book then places a tombstone - at least from the point of view of research - also on the concept of 'Autistic Spectrum' - on which the corresponding chapter of DSM5 was also based. The author affirms that it is an unproven theory that does not correspond to reality and that it ultimately prevents research because it maintains the basic errors that she described. The conclusion is that this diagnosis must be abandoned as a basis for research.

In her analysis the author uses the analogy of fever, which before was considered a disease in itself and only after the knowledge of many febrile diseases and the pathophysiological mechanisms involved was recognized as a symptom, not a disease. Similarly, autistic symptoms more or less associated with other symptoms are present in known diseases (although the pathogenetic pathway from the disease, e.g. the fragile X, to the symptom is unknown). The invitation that the author makes to the researchers is therefore to renounce the research of a common basis of autism and instead to focus on the possible brain alterations underlying the symptoms and the etiological agents that cause the alterations of the developing brain.

The book also does justice to a concept spread among insiders almost like a watchword of recognition, that of 'comorbidity', with which recent psychiatry explained the existence of different symptoms in the same individual, assuming that they were due to different diseases present simultaneously. Thus, epilepsy, intellectual disability, hyperactivity, which in many cases have been considered as diseases co-presenting autism, as different, entirely separate entities - precisely 'comorbidity', in modern psychiatric language - must be considered instead only as different symptoms present simultaneously.

Instead, a serious limitation of this book, typical of post-modern Anglo-Saxon researchers and their local epigones, one could say, - besides the sense of starting from a tabula rasa as if there had been nothing before them - is the scotomizing of relational, affective and emotional environmental aspects from the field of investigation of the possible factors involved. The author, addressing the possible environmental factors, examines extensively the theories of vaccinations, intestinal intolerances, heavy metals, etc., but dedicates only a few pages to psycho-social factors: he only quotes B Bettelheim and his affective theory, to bury with him any possibility of implication of environmental emotional factors in early life. Of all the modern psychological research on childhood he limits himself to mention the theories of attachment, which he does not go into in depth, with a superficiality that is astonishing compared to the amount of pages he has dedicated to the deepening of genetic 'biological' studies and also to 'physical' environmental factors. In this line he mentions only en passant the issue of autism in institutions, returned to the fore with studies on orphanages in Eastern Europe. He merely notes that autistic-like symptoms have been found in children in institutions and that these studies suggest that these children may have been adversely affected by the environment.

On these aspects one can almost perceive the existence of a taboo that seems to prevent the author and scholars like her from approaching these phenomena with a scientific method of observation and detection also of emotional and relational aspects. Such a scotomization of every possible relational environmental cause is astonishing. We think it is precisely the expression of the Manichean taboo that still pervades the Anglo-Saxon world and beyond, with regard to bio-psycho-social psychiatry and in particular psychoanalysis, considered devoid of any scientific value and thrown away together with its object of study, relationships and emotions, like the child together with bath water.

It remains, however, the merit of this book to make explicit the failure of at least twenty years of research and neurobiological theories on autism and to open a breach in the fortress of the autistic system that until now resists any methodological and substantial criticism. We hope that the breach will widen and may collapse this wall that, as was said, has been practically seized in the hands of some lobbies in the field of autism and related therapies. The effects produced on a generation of specialists are, however, disastrous, as many parents who found themselves in this situation have been able to verify. As in Andersen's fairy tale, perhaps, after the cry that 'the king is naked' people will no longer fear to recognize what they see with their own eyes and think with their own mind. In this way, we can go back to trying to understand each child individually with his or her experiences and in his or her environment, to look for possible obstacles and impediments to his or her development in all possible areas, not only organic-biological, but also psychological and environmental.

The Waterhouse book has been received very slowly and laboriously by the international scientific community, but progressively an important debate has developed (Appendix 1).

Chapter 6

Maybe autism doesn't exist

It is attributed to the English psychoanalyst and paediatrician D Winnicott, shortly after the 'discovery' of autism, the following statement: "The fate of autistic children became troubling the day Kanner isolated a syndrome he called Autism. From that day on, pediatricians stopped supporting a type of struggling mother: it was no longer necessary to speak to these poor troubled women, it became futile to remain supportive of their questions, since science had given the measure of its knowledge by putting a name to the disease"[12].

They seem to me prophetic words of what we are seeing today: parents who turn to pediatricians for some difficulty of their children and are immediately addressed to specialized services and centers where they are subjected to different visits by different specialists, tests, tables, measurements, etc., from the sum of which they are made a

---

[12] Winnicott D, Cit. in Brutti, Scotti, *Editoriale,* Quaderni di Psicoterapia Infantile, 1980, n3, pag12

statistical diagnosis with numbers and percentages and then given the good indication for all seasons: psychomotricity, speech therapy and aba, variously dosed and mixed.

The issue of autism has, in my view, reached a point where it can no longer be tolerated, because aspects of serious conceptual and scientific error are intricately mixed up with aspects that are perhaps fraudulent and manipulative and really dangerous to public health. In other words, for the welfare of children and families who are often overwhelmed at this time by sudden and wrong diagnoses that unnecessarily throw them into a hell of procedures, interventions, examinations and then diagnoses and therapies based on nothing.

Let's start with the current psychosis that has spread everywhere, which speaks of an epidemic of autism - or 'autism spectrum', we shall return to this in a moment - which, according to the latest epidemiological surveys, is estimated at 1 in every 38 children, more than 2% of the child population.

Twenty years ago it was 0.5 per thousand. There would therefore have been a huge increase in the number of cases in just a few years, which has led to a swarm of unproven explanatory hypotheses, such as vaccines or heavy metals, as well as the spread of panic and lobbying movements and miracle cures.

In fact, many people think that these epidemiological data are wrong, because they are based on basically incorrect findings, evaluation criteria and methods of diagnosis. They are data that spread alarm and disturbance in good or bad faith. There is probably a fundamental error, a

41

real conceptual and epistemological error, which we shall return to in a moment.

Meanwhile we note that not only from many parts outside the so-called 'scientific and academic world' dominant in recent years, but recently also from the inside there are criticism and rethinking that affect the whole building built by what have perhaps become real lobbies of autism. These criticisms question the very foundations, the very conceptual foundations of autism theory.

The entire conceptual construction of Autism was assembled by successive remakes until now. Before Kanner autistic children were not distinct from the amount of those considered simply mentally retarded, handicapped, 'degenerate', in a word in use in the first half of the twentieth century, and until forty years ago they were all more or less locked up in institutions. At the basis of the current conception of autism there is the assumption that the behaviors and symptoms observed in certain children must correspond to a brain disease or dysfunction that can account for the various symptoms. In this regard, the so-called Scientific Research on Autism - i.e. all the works published in the various scientific journals, presented at conferences of the scientific community, etc. - about twenty years ago has in practice restarted making tabula rasa of previous theories and knowledge. For twenty years it has spent a considerable amount of energy and funds in genetics, biochemistry, neurology, etc. in search of a unifying pathological basis that would account for all the disorders of children considered. The result seems to have been a total failure, as the aforementioned book *Rethinking Autism* by L Waterhouse acknowledges, which caused a stir in the environment.

In this regard, let us just remember that until 20 years ago only severely handicapped children were considered 'autistic'. In recent years even children with characteristics that are only slightly out of the average are diagnosed with 'autistic spectrum disorder'. This is due to the change in diagnostic methods, now based exclusively on the notorious tests that have entered into use everywhere that now almost no one is denied a diagnosis of 'autism spectrum'.

It is no longer a clinical diagnosis that globally reflects the serious impediment to everyday life that the conception of autism involved, but it is only a matter of assigning a place in the ranking, so to speak. Above a certain numerical level, let's say 10, the diagnostic algorithm allows to enter the first drawer of the 'spectrum', above another level, let's say 20, to enter a further drawer, and then another one. In all there are three drawers (like the three cards), with Slight, Medium and Severe labels, in the chest of drawers called Autistic Spectrum Disorder.

Let me make some analogies to better describe the situation.

It has always come spontaneously to me the comparison with the cough, for example, where one could create a 'Tuberculosis Spectrum' (much more easily than looking for the bacterium responsible), which above 10 coughs allows to be put in the Mild drawer, above 20 in the Medium one and above 30 in the Severe one. With good peace of mind for Dr Koch and the microbiological immunological X-ray blood tests etc. which are the basis of the scientific medical diagnosis of tuberculosis, as well as the clinical evaluation.

Another analogy can be a cycling or running race, where at various points of the route the time of the participants is taken, and according to the delays they are divided into various groups, and are considered to be 'Severe', 'Medium' or 'Slightly Slow'... The times taken usually are not indicative of pathologies.

To make another analogy: many people leave for their holidays by car at the beginning of summer. Some of them do not arrive at their destination and encounter different problems at different stages of the journey that delay or prevent them from travelling. But there is not a disease called 'aut(omobil)ism' that manifests itself between the holidaymakers blocking those at the beginning and those later on. There are different obstacles: who punctures a tire, who burns the engine, who burns the carburetor, who misses the road, who is without petrol... Maybe at a certain point some people stop, get out of the car, rave, get angry and maybe they go crazy and do other strange things. But they don't have an identical disease or some 'spectrum' of diseases with similar and different symptoms. They have simply encountered different and common accidents and obstacles on their way that may have slowed them down and then made them angry and freaked out.

So it is for children who begin their vital journey and at a certain point encounter obstacles that slow them down or stop them or divert them. Maybe they get nervous and freak out and start making strange movements, sometimes... It makes little sense to look for a common disease responsible for all the detours, much more sense to try to assist the 'travelers' by intervening immediately to help them in case of accidents or other anomalies and allow them to get back on the road without losing too much time or getting lost or going back.

Twenty years of medical biochemical genetic biochemical research, therefore, have not led to the slightest valid confirmation of what is still pompously said and written everywhere: 'Autism is a neurobiological disease'. There is no proof of this. The mountain has not given birth to the slightest mouse, but only an amount of printed paper that even in the evaluations of the 'independent' agencies of control and evaluation of scientific publications, such as the Cochrane Collaboration, receives for the most part ratings of inadequacy in terms of method and scientific credibility [13].

Not only that. In the concept of 'autism' and 'autistic spectrum' it becomes increasingly clear that the most diverse situations have been mixed and it is therefore in this soup or salad of 'data' that we have tried to find the skein.

What can we say about the therapies that are now distributed like rain: they are simply done blindly, on nonexistent 'diseases' of which nothing has been understood. For the most part they are paid by families, but there are

---

[13]Reichow B, Hume K, Barton EE, Boyd BA. *Early intensive behavioral intervention (EIBI) for young children with autism spectrum disorders (ASD),* Cochrane Database of Systematic Reviews 2018, Issue 5. Art. No.: CD009260. DOI: 10.1002/14651858.CD009260.pub3.
(Even Cochrane Coll., however, does not wonder about the validity of the diagnosis of autism itself).

strong drives to make public services and states pay, to spread a certain type of intervention even more.

Perhaps there is a basic conceptual error in the whole issue from the outset. From Kanner onwards, those who came afterwards have dealt with "autism" as an entity in itself, without in the least questioning its existence. Kanner's proposal to consider children with certain symptoms as affected by an entity called Early Childhood Autism was immediately accepted by all, even with D Winnicott's prophetic commentary. Everyone accepted the idea of a disease of which 'autistic' symptoms were considered an effect, but no one cared to prove its existence.

These children were then called 'autistic' and were given essential symptoms and accessories to diagnose them. And then similar symptoms were recognized, considered as 'autistic traits', under different conditions from more classical cases. Finally, indicators and detectors of asymptomatic or almost asymptomatic cases ('below the threshold') were identified, thus extending the field of casuistry more and more. In this way, more and more different cases were collected in a single whole, the Autistic Spectrum: the unique cauldron that Kanner had feared was thus realized.

But the risk is that this entity does not actually exist, since no actual reality has ever been demonstrated and it is in fact an abstract construct, a concept, a 'ghost' or a real 'spectrum', as the word itself suggests in the Italian language, to which a real object does not correspond. A more mystical-theological than scientific field, in the end.

On the other hand, there are children and their families who find obstacles and difficulties in following their developmental path so that they accumulate 'delays' in the planned route, or sometimes 'deviations' from the road considered 'normal', or common. I have the impression that dealing with 'autism' and the theories that have been built to 'explain' it, has long prevented us from seeing these children in their development and the factors that could and may hinder it. Almost like the medieval philosophy that dealt with abstract categories, with great diatribes about supernatural transcendent characteristics, and which has long prevented us from seeing real natural phenomena again in a scientific and not dogmatic way.

Let us try to retrace the history of this error.

The conceptual error of autism

Psychiatry has tried to follow the medical model of disease as emerged in Western medicine in recent centuries, based essentially on the linear principle of cause-effect, an injury - a disease. In this it has been followed in the last century by a part of psychology that has been dominant in recent decades, which has come to renounce the suffix 'psycho-' in its name: cognitive sciences. So perhaps it has moved away from the human to approach the mechanical, computer sciences.

The medical model of the disease is based on the following points, in an extreme synthesis: Symptoms and signs → diagnostic hypothesis of injury or damaging process → instrumental confirmation → therapy established by scientific evidence. Example I – symptoms (fever, sore throat, rash) → diagnosis: scarlet fever → confirmation by microbiological immunological blood tests → therapy: antibiotics. Example II - symptoms(epileptic seizure, headache, neurological objective signs, ocular fundus edema) → diagnosis: expansive brain process (tumor) → confirmation by instrumental examinations → therapy: medical radiological surgery.

Despite the hopes, however, in psychiatry in the vast majority of cases it has not been possible to follow the medical model, except in the use of the gown, of the language for insiders, in the bureaucratic organization, in the association disease-drugs.This is because the symptoms (behavior), with few exceptions, could not be associated with instrumental, biochemical, anatomical confirmations of lesions of organs and their possible causes. The exceptions are precisely those cases in which neurological symptoms are added to certain psychiatric symptoms and the tests confirm the presence of inflammatory, dysmetabolic or tumor pathological processes, etc. In the majority of cases, even after years and decades of 'illness' (or 'disorder', a term used in psychiatry to escape the obligations of the medical model that requires the instrumental verification and demonstration of etiopathogenesis while maintaining the advantages of attributing the cause of the disorders to a given entity, without having to take care to prove their existence), no significant evidence of a brain damaging process to which the symptoms can be attributed is found, not even at an autopsy level.

Therapies in these cases started blindly, from the random discovery of coarse pharmacological effects on symptoms (sedation, excitement) and the development of drugs similar to those discovered by chance. The possible etiopathogenetic hypotheses, the most famous being that of 'biochemical brain imbalance', have disappeared without trace, it would seem.

Something similar happened with so-called autism. A poorly defined concept, from time immemorial, between symptom and 'syndrome' (i.e. a set of symptoms whose relationship is not well known) has at some point been attributed the value of 'disease'. In this way it has been possible to attribute to it the cause of autistic symptoms, in a magic circle that has produced the statement that can be read in every treatise of recent years: "autism is a neurobiological disorder whose causes are not yet known". As if to say: "autism is the cause of autism". Absurd and tautological, therefore, but according to the agreement of all the official 'authorities' on the subject it is definitely something neurobiological in nature. "Ipse dixit", it was said in the days of Scholasticism. The human being himself is neurobiological in nature, on the other hand, and the progressive extension of the criteria of inclusion of the 'autistic spectrum' is proceeding towards comprehending the whole of humanity in what will then become the 'human spectrum'.

The myth of autism

The concept of autism, therefore, taken up with the meaning of a specific clinical picture by the child psychiatrist Kanner in 1943, has had great success and has become a huge and so to speak useful thing for all seasons. From this moment on, everyone, among clinicians and researchers of the most diverse tendencies and orientations, psychiatrists, psychologists, psychoanalysts, educators, etc., has taken it up for their own purposes and used it according to their interests and needs. Reading the articles and books of the 60s and 70s of the last century, we find described cases of 'autistic' children who are very different from each other, often incongruous even within the different currents and schools of psychiatry and psychoanalysis.

No one wondered if this entity really existed or tried to prove its existence, but everyone tried to find its core, which - apart from unbalanced neurotransmitters or 'mirror neurons' perhaps broken - for some was the 'autistic state of mind', for others the 'lack of a theory of the mind', or hypersensitivity to stimuli, etc., etc.. The existence of 'autism' was always taken for granted, beyond the need for evidence of the existence of this entity.

It was affirmed in the early days that the definition of "autism" had made it possible to differentiate this type of children from all the others with whom they were previously mixed, in institutions, that is, children and people with disabilities of various kinds, mental deficiencies, traumas, infections, etc., etc. It was thought that this would allow great progress in the search for causes and therapies.

However, a chaos prevailed in which everyone saw his or her own 'autism' in a true and proper Babel that will well remember those who attended conferences and publications in those years. It was in order to overcome the confusion and the difficulty of comparison between the different clinicians that the American revisionist wave of statistical diagnostic psychiatry, which produced the various DSM 3, 4, 4R, began in the 80's, trying to establish a common basis for the definition of psychiatric diagnoses. Dissatisfaction with the results gradually led to new changes that eventually, in the DSM5, led to the reunification of almost all cases of developmental alterations into a single category, the Autistic Spectrum, returning to the confusion and undifferentiation of the period prior to the discovery or invention of autism. The presence of some similar symptoms leads to put all in the same cauldron, even if a number of other characteristics are completely different.

All this is always without the slightest instrumental evidence of a documented basic neurobiological or neurophysiologic alteration.

So giving a name to the thing obtained by putting together some signs and symptoms and characteristics has created an entity that has immediately had, so to speak, an autonomous life and that has become the object of research and studies aimed at describing its attributes and qualities and seeking its manifestations in the various ways in which they could appear. Clinicians and researchers have in every way tried to define its characteristics and modes of functioning by collecting and classifying its manifestations in increasingly refined ways and trying to recognize them even if they were variously camouflaged in living beings. But all this does not constitute a clear proof of the existence of that entity and shows that the question has remained at a mythological-theological level rather than at a scientific level.

The conclusion of this discourse is that perhaps autism does not exist, but everyone has always believed it existed and behaved accordingly. A bit like the fairy tale of the Clothes of the Emperor of Andersen: as is known only a child had the spontaneity, not to say the courage and the imprint, to shout that the king was naked.

We should therefore perhaps forget the term autism, because it is misleading and at this point more harmful than useful: it gives the false idea that we know the reason for certain phenomena, while admitting that the causes are not yet scientifically known. Let me say that It is a worse remedy than the hole (the lack of knowledge): it simply shifts the matter to higher planes, so to speak, leaving to the lower planes the task of exercising magical and ritual practices. It seems to me a situation similar to when men thought they knew the reason for the lightning: it was Jupiter who threw them and the priests were deputies for the rites and sacrifices to appease their anger.

As we know in the history of civilization, mythical-religious explanations precede scientific knowledge but often persist indefinitely. The so-called diagnosis of 'Autism', which so much now occupies the experts and terrorizes families, risks being a mythical-religious explanation that does not help our knowledge, but merely reassures - paradoxically - people and 'experts' themselves instead of admitting that they do not know. As was once said about mental illness, even autism is perhaps actually a myth. As in the myths of ancient times, the myth also has the function of justifying a certain state of affairs by proclaiming its divine origin, or in this case 'scientific', using science in an absolutely improper way, whereas there is no real justification for such a state of affairs.

Obviously there are people with difficulties of mental development and we need terms to describe them and understand their difficulties and help them cope with their disabilities. But the terms 'autism', 'autistic', etc. have now become charged with too many mystifying meanings and it would be good at this point to give them up and replace them with others that do not prevent people from seeing things. Especially in childhood, which is now being affected together with families by the serious nightmare of the Autistic System.

Children with developmental difficulties and their families need help to deal with the problems they encounter. However, they need not 'autism specialists' but 'development specialists' who have the necessary skills for any medical, psychological and relational aspects that may be involved. The same specialists, on the other hand, should also be in play to follow the development of children with known and documented neurological and other diseases that give developmental difficulties and sometimes disabilities and handicaps of various degrees. On the other hand, neurological syndromes that are now recognized, such as Rett's syndrome and Landau-Kleffner syndrome, among others, have gradually detached themselves from the cauldron of autism and are now among the diseases that can give symptoms similar to those considered 'autistic' and consequent disabilities. Using the mechanical-quantitative diagnostic criteria in use, they would still be included in the autistic spectrum.

This type of developmental specialist has, in my opinion, disappeared[14] at the moment in both public and private services dealing with children, replaced by 'technical' experts in specific but limited areas who do not have the necessary overall clinical expertise. This expertise is not made up of the sum of so many limited skills, as has been the prevailing model in recent decades which has led precisely to sectorialization, the loss of global skills and the situation that these families often experience when they turn to existing services.

It is likely that this problem will have growing repercussions in the near future, with the exit of the medical and health care personnel trained in the 1970s - 1980s, who had a broad and wide-ranging vision of both medical and psychosocial problems of development and mental life, progressively replaced by personnel with more mechanical and sectorial training. This is, on the other hand, something that is already affecting all medicine and the health and social organization of our time

---

[14]These considerations apply to the current Italian situation. I do not know if they can be valid for other countries as well.

Chapter 7

New optics, new conceptual tools

The possible conceptual error made so far with regard to autism and the autistic spectrum (the effects of which are discussed in these pages) has perhaps depended on the application to the observed phenomena, i.e. the alteration of psychological development and the presence of behavioral anomalies, of the linear logical model used for physical diseases and their symptoms, typical of positivistic western medicine: symptom - organ alteration - disease (lesion, genetic). In genetics dominated the model Gene - Enzyme (altered) - Disease.

Probably, instead, the phenomena of development and behavior, in their great complexity, variability and dependence on different factors not easily knowable, are better understood using the tools of non-linear logic, developed in mathematics in the theories of chaos and complexity. For some time now, the application of these new mathematical models has been affecting different fields, from meteorology, economics, population studies, liquid flows, etc. The applications of chaos theory are also found in fields such as biomedical sciences, psychology, development and functioning of the mind[15]. This field of mathematics has had very interesting developments, methods have been developed to analyze phenomena that could not be studied before because they are interested in unpredictable variables and unknown starting points. Concepts and tools have been developed to define them, such as non-linear equations, attraction points, butterfly effect, etc.[16] Applying this viewpoint to psychic development and its events we can perhaps make interesting observations that could move developmental psychology, which has become bogged down in so-called autistic phenomena with no apparent way out.

From this point of view, psychic development can be seen as the flow of a fluid - after all, the hydraulic model and the electromagnetic and corpuscular (quantum) electromagnetic model are widely present also in biology - which can have a regular, 'laminar', obstacle-free tendency, or rather a 'turbulent' one, as when it encounters obstacles that create turbulence, eddies, anomalous waves, in short, a chaotic trend.

Probably it can help us to make a connection between the Florence flood and the difficulties of psychic development. What's that got to do with it? It could be said. Just a moment of patience.

The flooding of Florence - a rare event but repeated every century or so - depends on the convergence of differ-

[15] Society for Chaos Theory, *Nonlinear Dynamics in Psychology and Life Science,* http://www.societyforchaostheory.org/home/
[16] Ischi, Carini, Gardini, Tenti – *Sulle orme del caos* – Bruno Mondadori

ent factors, including the abnormal amount of occasional rain along its course and the presence of the Ponte Vecchio at the point where the river is narrowest, almost in the centre of the city. The areas of the city near the bridge are partially down level, i.e. lower than the banks. If a flood drags with it abundant debris, including branches, tree trunks, etc., it is easy for debris to collect at the pylons of the bridge and for the aisles to be obstructed, so as to create a dam that blocks the flow of water and quickly overflows into the surrounding streets, with the serious and tragic effects that have been seen.

The same thing can happen in psychic development, which normally follows a fairly established average course, so to speak a regular, linear flow. But different obstacles can be created that cause disturbances to the 'flow', which can thus become turbulent and chaotic under certain circumstances, due to the often random combination of different factors. In this way, sometimes a stop of the flow (developmental blockage) and, so to speak, a flood invading the surrounding territory (anomalous behavior) can occur. These terms can describe what happens in psychic development, where often different obstacles create 'turbulences' that alter the linear, orderly flow, leading to complete or almost complete blocks during development with overflow and outflow of altered and disturbing behavior.

This descriptive model does not need to pose symptom-disease-type equations, or rather these can be understood in broader concepts that see different causal factors, some of which are unknown, that contribute to determining similar phenomena. Rather than on the causes, for the moment unknowable, interventions should focus on the nodal points where to intervene to restore a situation of 'fluidity'. A bit like it happens, to use another analogy, in traffic jams where the specific causes often remain indeterminate, while structural situations can be evaluated on which to intervene with appropriate modifications.

In order to get out of the current impasse of research, clinic and aid interventions in developmental disorders, it is therefore necessary, in my opinion, to get out of the purely linear concept that has dominated in medicine and psychology until now, to free oneself from prejudices and taboos in order to face and find new tools for observation and analysis of very complex and often chaotic phenomena such as those of psychic development and behavior.

The linear medical-biological model (which recites its axiom as if it were the first of the ten commandments: autism is a neurobiological disorder of genetic origin...) has imposed itself also because of the difficulty of dealing with environmental aspects, not so much the toxic infectious ones etc., as the human relational ones.

In the early epochs of observation of 'autistic' phenomena many initial statements attributed to Kanner and Bettelheim were probably unnecessarily blaming the parents. Extrapolated from the contexts they became slogans (the clichés of 'refrigerated mothers', cold intellectual parents, etc.) used against 'environmentalist' positions, so to speak. As a reaction, many have gone on to deny, scotomize, not even take into consideration the possible presence of inadequate, dysfunctional, disturbing aspects for development, in the environmental modalities of care, organization, relationship and in the experiences made by the child, aspects that cannot be excluded a priori in any case, if not by ideological choice. We have a paradigmatic demonstration of the importance of environmental factors in cases of so-called institutional autism, once frequent (see Appendix 5), where known environmental factors are associated with alterations in development and behavior that are reversible up to a certain point if environmental conditions were changed. In fact, a wrong 'moralistic' and blameworthy position has been opposed by an ideological position that is equally wrong, equally moralistic but of absolute opposite sign. That position has tried to eliminate the problem by eliminating environmental research tout-court, always maintaining a 'Holy Inquisition' perspective and not a scientific position.

It is not the possible shortcomings of the parents - possible in any context: nobody is perfect, as every parent knows, if not too narcissistic - to be guilty of children's disorders, but these can be one of the competing factors that determine the problems, often modifiable if focused. To get rid of the blaming positions of the early days of investigating these aspects, one 'threw the baby (that is the environment) out with the bath water', and got lost in an inextricable maze, because it became impossible to see anything with the blinkers and darkened lenses worn so far by researchers conditioned by the surrounding climate. Research on autism has given up dealing with the emotional and relational environmental conditions in which children live and so it practically blinds itself by cutting away a good part of the reality it should deal with.

On the contrary, science and research on the causes of children's developmental difficulties has everything to gain from the possibility to get rid of these impediments in order to observe more openly the phenomena we are facing and try to focus on their various aspects. We would probably have more tools for intervention and help and rehabilitation in the difficult situations we are dealing with.

Chapter 8

The refusal syndromes

In the context of the behavioral manifestations that the child neuropsychiatrist or psychiatrist is often called upon to deal with, there are situations that seem to be characterized by a conscious refusal on the part of the person concerned to adapt to social demands typical of different ages. This refusal often puts the subject at odds with family members and institutions, and sometimes evokes the use of psychiatric diagnoses to explain and 'cure' his behavior. A name for these situations could be 'refusal syndromes'.

At different ages, this behavior takes on different aspects. In adulthood, for example, we find people who at some point isolate themselves from their social context, leaving their jobs, families and often literally disappear without being found any more. This is dealt with on broadcasts such as 'Who has seen the missing person', etc. There are quite famous cases, around which more or less mysterious and fictionalized stories have arisen, such as that of the Italian nuclear physicist Ettore Majorana, who disappeared at the end of the thirties, on whom the Italian writer Leonardo Sciascia wrote a short novel, or the Italian economist Federico Caffè, who disappeared suddenly from today to tomorrow in the '80s of the last century.

Once, perhaps even nowadays, some people abandoned the life they had lived until then to retire to convents; on the other hand, monastic life could attract men and women not only for religious vocation or other reasons but also for the withdrawal from the world that it involved or allowed.

Other people radically changed their lives at a certain point in their evolution, or went on long journeys that took them out of their usual environment. Here too, the possible motivations include a refusal of the situation quo ante. Up to now these behaviors have not yet been labeled by psychiatry with diagnoses related to some brain pathology. In others, however, this has not been the case.

We cannot forget the refusal to live which is one of the motivations of suicide, an act generally considered psychiatric in nature but which today is accepted in various parts as a conscious choice to which the social organization of certain states provides support and assistance.

In recent years, the attention of the media, as well as insiders, has been attracted by the condition of young adults or late-adolescents who literally lock themselves in their homes, in their rooms. They were first described in Japan, hence the Japanese term Hikikomori by which they are known. They refuse social contact with anyone, often limiting themselves to allowing their mother to pass their food through a narrow opening in a doorway left ajar. A total withdrawal from outside life made possible perhaps by the somewhat condescending family environment. I have seen several of these situations over the years, almost all of them extremely difficult to know and extremely difficult to solve. Other situations of a less extreme degree, but with avoidance of social relationships and very limited life, are defined as 'social phobia', when they are not associated with other symptoms that lead to more serious diagnoses.

We also find a component of refusal in situations described in other contexts, where there are family and cultural conflicts. They are in some ways controversial in interpretation, but they are certainly part of the individual and group psychological field. They are the so-called Syndromes of Parental Alienation and Cultural Alienation ((not accepted by everyone), in which a boy or girl suddenly rejects a parent or the whole family, accused of abuse and violence, and tries to break all contact with the rejected, resisting strenuously to any attempt to change the situation created. I will not go into the motivations on which there are strong disagreements between the insiders.

Still in adolescence we cannot forget to mention the rejection of food, which represents the most striking and characteristic manifestation of mental anorexia.

Another similar behavior, at a younger age, at the time of elementary or middle school, characterized by refusal - a term that also appears in the diagnostic definition that psychiatrists and child psychologists make - is 'school refusal', or 'school phobia'. This condition sees boys and girls without any particular learning problems gradually or suddenly refusing to go to school, without any obvious reasons related to the school environment. One can often find, deepening the knowledge of these cases, situations of intra-family difficulties that create a great sense of insecurity for the child, such as a parent's illness or something else, that lead him to not want to leave the house, almost for fear of not finding it when he returns, or to find unpleasant changes.

At the same age we often find situations and behaviors characterized by the refusal to adapt to social rules and limits and the authority of adults. Such situations, which often create serious turmoil in schools, are now diagnosed as 'oppositional-provocative disorders'.

Going backwards in age, in kindergarten, one finds children who do not speak at school or outside the family environment, even though they speak well in the family. Again, this behavior seems to express a refusal, in this case too, to express themselves in spoken language, while they often adhere to proposed activities and are more or less available to non-verbal communication. The diagnosis coined by psychiatrists for these cases was of 'elective mutism', then modified into 'selective' mutism, for some reason, going from emphasizing the 'choice' (from the Latin 'eligere', choose) not to speak, to 'selecting' the situations in which the child speaks or not. Perhaps it is to deny that it is a conscious 'choice', preferring to think of a less conscious and determined behavior, evoked by 'selected' environments.

Finally, at even younger ages, in the second and third years of life, and here we come to the subject that interests us, it happens to see children who limit their interest and their relationship to objects, toys, etc., which they use appropriately, but completely avoiding having to deal with people. They are children who often show normal understanding and intelligence but tend not to have contact with others and do not communicate or speak.

A further step is that of children who are not interested in either people or objects, except in a limited and often atypical way, do not use objects and people according to their function, but use them in idiosyncratic ways, as a means to reach something out of their reach or to fill their time. These children seem to refuse contact and withdraw from social life and even from things in the world, showing no interest and avoiding or reacting with irritation to attempts to involve them. They are those who were once mostly diagnosed as 'autistic'. Now as we know the autistic spectrum has extended its dominance to much larger territories.

All the behaviors described above are characterized by refusal and to varying degrees by withdrawal from the social environment. The consequences can be very different, depending on the age at which rejection occurs. Adults usually maintain matured global abilities while subjects in the developmental age may be not able to learn new abilities and to lose acquired skills. Children of very few years of age may not acquire most of the skills that depend on social interaction, such as the language and the ability to adapt and cope with different situations in daily life, thus creating vicious circles of non-learning and increased isolation.

The situations described have almost all been somehow reduced to psychiatric pathologies, with different diagnoses, from *Hikikomori* (still missing a 'western' diagnosis), to social phobia, school phobia, elective-selective mutism, etc... In very young children there was talk first of 'autism' and then of 'autistic spectrum', with which perhaps more problems were created - terminological, diagnostic, epidemiological - than those they wanted to solve.

Anyone who has had contact and experience of relations with so-called autistic children - not only at the level of compiling tests or performing score calculations - has often been faced with the refusal of the child and his or her strenuous resistance to being involved in some way in a relationship or sharing. The child who dedicates himself - in a way appropriate to his age - to games and objects, but rejects and avoids involvement with people with impassive expression, gives the idea of a somewhat conscious choice to avoid this kind of experience, i.e. the relationship with a person.

How to account for apparently so different ways of reacting at different ages, but with such similar characteristics? Brain and cellular lesions, biochemical alterations that cause a reaction of refusal and withdrawal? Perhaps there are other possible explanations, one at the level of normal psychological development, the other at the phylogenetic level.

In the normal psychic development, it should be remembered that we find a behavior similar to what is described above even in different situations, not pathological, but physiological and characteristic of a phase of development, the so-called 'stranger reaction'. It is known to anyone caring for children that towards the end of the first year of life the child shows distrust, rejection and avoidance if he comes into contact with an unknown person, and this becomes marked discomfort and weeping if he does not find comfort in a family member close to him. At this stage of psychological development the child rejects the stranger and automatically turns to the mother or the person he knows for protection and consolation. It is also the time of difficulty in detachment and separation from the known person, which is a universal manifestation of children in the first days of entering the nursery, unless this occurs before the eighth or ninth month when the child is not yet fully able to grasp the detachment and the difference between family members and strangers.

The reaction to strangers is a physiological manifestation in the development of children, useful phylogenetically to the defense of the species, with attachment to known people and distrust and estrangement from unknown ones.

Sometimes a child can have this attitude even after the age of the reaction to the stranger, at the beginning of acquaintance with a new person in certain circumstances. In fact, such an attitude is ubiquitous even in adults, more or less manifestly. Almost all children, for example in the examination room with the doctor, are at first cautious and suspicious, but then they check the situation and if they feel safe and comfortable they sometimes develop very quickly and very clearly during the examination, often becoming openly familiar with the person they have come into contact with and enjoying a meaningful relational experience. At other times the child evolves positively during the session only over a long period of time, while others still cannot overcome the initial distrust, thus showing various difficulties in his psychological development. The evolution in the first session thus gives an opportunity to make useful evaluations, also prognostically.

Moving on to the phylogenetic level, i.e. the global evolution of living beings, it is known that at a primitive level - on the biological scale but also on the scale of civilization - the most typical reaction in the face of a situation of danger, alarm, unknown, extraneous, is the so-called 'fight-flight'. It seems that the subject has only the alternative of attacking or fleeing, depending on the power relations of the moment. Before this there is, perhaps, even more primitive, the reaction of immobility, of mimicry with the environment, in order not to be seen by the predator. With respect to the reaction of fight-flight I can think of some children who show an aggressive behavior and beat, bite, scratch their peers and also adults, without showing fear and even challenging reprimands and punishments or even 'beating', with the typical challenge phrase 'you did nothing to me'... That these children for some reason implement the solution of the attack, between the two possible options?

But, apart from these children, it is understandable that at certain levels of age, ability and maturity perhaps the only alternative available may be escape, refusal, withdrawal and avoidance, because power relations, so to speak, are too unfavorable. So that to withdraw, to avoid contact, to refuse to respond, in a situation perceived as dangerous, may be a clear 'choice', even if it may be difficult to accept that such a small child makes it, as a mother once commented in front of the evident behavior of her child in an observational session.

This hypothesis is instead less difficult to understand and accept in older children, adolescents and adults, where it does not seem deniable that it is a choice, perhaps forced, even if someone will find the most varied explanations to include these behaviors in genetically and biochemically determined behaviors...

Immobility and mimicry could be observed with a certain frequency in asylums and institutions of a few decades ago, where an inpatient could flatten against the wall or stand motionless on a tile for hours, without anyone taking care of him, until he was no longer seen.

At the moment we have no reliable explanation of the behaviors described. However, we cannot exclude that they manifest themselves in reaction to experiences perceived as negative, of discomfort, of danger; in other words, they are somehow linked to experiences lived. From some situations seen more closely, it seems that such reactions can quickly impose themselves as habits, which over time become almost automatic and difficult to change.

The reaction to the stranger, mentioned above, seems strongly evocative as a paradigmatic model of reaction to an uncomfortable situation, triggered by the perception of strangeness as dangerous in some way. Linked to the typical reaction to separation from the parent, to kindergarten or other occasions, it usually lasts a limited period and is overcome by the child in its development. But sometimes it persists much longer and creates the basis for a diffident, 'shy' and somehow reluctant attitude to face new experiences, which is usually considered a personality aspect, 'character', as they say, and not a specific pathology (maybe for a little longer...).

The experience of the stranger and that of separation are, on the other hand, inevitable experiences in today's reality; we can think that in other eras and in other latitudes there could be fixed and unchanging environments in which these experiences did not occur. Surely the modern social organization in the Western world - with nuclear families, kindergartens, life regulated in some way according to social, work, etc. needs and not individual, family, 'child-friendly' ones etc. - can account for an accentuation of such reactions and the spread that the manifestations described above seem to have in recent times, culminating with the so called epidemic of autism that many people claim to occur.

In adult, adolescent and late childhood manifestations - i.e. from Hikikomori to social phobia to school phobias to elective mutism - it is so far uncontested that these are psychological, perhaps relational and family problems. On the other hand, in early childhood manifestations, which are usually tested all 'within the autistic spectrum', if not in autism *tout-court,* it is unusual to talk about psychological, relational and family problems, while the dogma of the genetic biological cause, although still unknown, dominates.

While waiting for future research, perhaps appropriately amended and reorganized, to give more convincing results than it has done so far and to clarify the possible causes and remedies, it is worth - given the extent of the stakes, the whole mental development of the person - to return to deal with the experiences that children make in their environment, so as to better understand the possible reasons for their reactions. The approach to children characterized by these modes of refusal, distrust and withdrawal should become an all-round approach, a work to be done together with the families to eventually find out if their children react to some uncomfortable situation, maybe not recognized, maybe 'normal' but excessive for the sensitivities of that child in that given moment. What is at stake is the possibility to get them back on a path of development that allows the maturation of their global mental capacities. The proposed work should not be the repetitive and stereotyped obligatory trinomial 'psychomotricity-logopedia-behavioral therapy', - but an approach aimed at helping parents and their children to face possible difficulties, just what Winnicott saw disappearing, regretting, for the discovery of 'autism'.

Child psychiatrists and psychologists should return to dealing specifically with normal and altered childhood development and conditions that may favor or hinder it.

Chapter 9

Vital impulse and developmental disorders.

Interest, curiosity, desire to know.

The authors who have dealt with psychic development agree on attributing the development of all living beings to an innate evolutionary drive. With different names
(élan vital, vital impulse, life drive, etc., Montessori,
Vigotsky, Freud, Darwin, etc., not least Dante with his
"Love that moves the world and the other stars") all, religious and lay, see the development of all living beings as
the fruit of a life force that would act in nature as the engine of development of every living being according to a
programming, so to speak, species-specific, based, we now
know, on the genetic code that contains the potential for
species-specific development. On the other hand, we know
that every living being, of the animal or vegetable king-
dom, develops the characteristics and abilities proper to its
species on the basis of the encounter between its innate en-
dowment and the surrounding environment, which provides
the essential elements, such as nutrition and environmental
conditions, etc., for the realization of the potentialities pre-

sent in nuce in the individual. Nature (genotype) and culture (environmental conditions) both contribute to the manifestations (phenotype) that we observe in individuals, be they animals, trees or people.

We see at work this evolutionary drive in the child (and in the adult) in the form of interest, curiosity, desire, and careful observation can capture the differences between the different individuals.

Why do some young children show interest and curiosity and desire to know, to get in touch and communicate and, at the same age and apparently with similar abilities, others do not? Excluding situations of mental retardation, sensory disorders, epilepsy, etc., there are often no brain causes to motivate these differences. Excluding also conditions of visual and auditory sensory deficits, and seriously deficient environmental conditions such as those seen in cases of 'institutional autism', is it possible that less dramatic and obvious environmental causes are the cause? Can there be environmental conditions that facilitate and stimulate curiosity and interest and desire expressions of innate vitality, and others that hinder them? On these aspects it seems to me that psychological and psychiatric research has been very lacking in recent decades. Fortunately, recently there has been a resumption of studies on the effects on the brain, both functional and anatomical, of early life experiences, in particular of negative environmental events, such as neglect and abuse [17]. The results

---

[17] C H Zeanah, K. L. Humphreys, *Child Abuse and Neglect*, JAACAP 2018,57,9,637

seem particularly promising [18]. The research on human environmental factors, kicked out the door, came back through the window, trying not to make too much noise.

It is clear that desires and curiosity are encouraged by gratification and ease of access to appropriate stimuli, and then by motivation, which can also overcome obstacles and difficulties, as in those who do not hesitate to launch themselves to the conquest of Everest. But this comes later. At the beginning, availability, ease of access and gratification are probably the most important aspects that reinforce or discourage the vital thrust. Those who succeed in an attempt will tend to move forward in exploration, those who fail, after a few attempts will abandon the game, research, etc..

So the lack of success in the attempts made, but also the lack of opportunities, of availability, of possibilities of experience, the difficulty of having access to them and the lack of gratification can be factors hindering the cognitive drive. Those who do not have a bicycle do not learn how to use it, those who do not have a river or pool, etc., do not learn to swim. But even those who have one and don't throw themselves into it... It is well known that the great climber and explorer Reinhold Messner cannot swim. Those who do not have a sea to experience will not learn to swim in it. If the water doesn't fit, the duck doesn't float, says an Italian adage.

---

[18]J L Luby, *Editorial: The primacy of parenting*, J. Child Psychology and Psychiatry, April 2020, 61,4

Is it possible that in the face of conditions in which cognitive experiences have been poorly fostered there could be at some point a renunciation, a withdrawal from attempts, out of excessive frustration? Some children show a, it is said, low tolerance to frustration and tend to give up the first obstacles after a few attempts. Is it possible that this condition, frequently observed and reported by families and teachers etc., is not so much an innate, genetic basis (as biological psychology tends to think), but a point of arrival of previous frustrated and frustrating experiences, after which at a certain point the child renounces to continue trying? At least we can maintain the doubt.

Observing certain children you can see how a dichotomy, a split of their curiosity, interest and desire: on the one hand a normal or almost normal curiosity and interest in objects, games and environments, on the other almost no interest and curiosity for people, for getting in touch and communicating. Will there be some 'mirror neuron' or similar that differentiates inanimate objects from animated ones? Or could it be possible that for these children it was easier to deal with objects than with people, because the former are and have been easy to access, know and foresee, while people have been much less so, for different reasons? Could it be that there is a limit, a threshold to the tolerance of frustration in the relationship with people and that the child therefore above this threshold desists from the interest for a part of the world, the human one, to keep it for the one of things, easier to know? But the thresholds, such as those of tolerance to pain, fatigue, etc., also depend on experience, habit, training.

This raises the question of evaluating the quality of experience, and not only the quantity, made available to a child for his or her growth. Not unlike in the area of food, where today there seems to be a lot of sensitivity to the quality of food - even if a part of the world still has the problem of quantity and hunger - there should also be a similar sensitivity to the quality of experiences that a child may need in the area of psychological growth. Insufficient and 'bad' nutrition (physical and mental) can have negative consequences for growth and health (physical and mental).

In the field of psychic development and mental health we still know very little about the quality of useful and necessary experiences and possible 'toxic' or unfavorable aspects. The never enough cited observations of children who grew up in orphanages and then were adopted show how the lack of certain experiences or the 'toxic' aspects of those experiences can be negative for the development and health of children.

A cross-eyed developmental science has so far dealt almost exclusively with measuring performance and looking for cellular biological, biochemical and genetic characteristics behind the difficulties of development and mental health. It has not dealt with human environmental conditions. This serious deficiency needs to be filled, returning to the observations of Montessori[19], Vigotsky[20] and others, who have somehow been isolated and relegated to the educational pedagogical context and expelled from the psychiatric psychological one, at least in my experience.

---

[19] Montessori, Maria (1948). *The Discovery of the Child.* Madras, Kalakshetra,
[20] Vygotsky L S, (1934), *Thought and Language*, The MIT Presse

It seems therefore fundamental to give new vigor to studies and psychological research on child development, on the one hand, at the educational and research level, and on the other, at the care level, to add to what is done today by pediatricians etc. in developmental screening, the necessary elements of attention to the global environmental situation of the child. Not only or not so much therefore evaluate performance with the various fashionable tests, but evaluate the environments around the individual child so that they can eventually be provided with the 'water' that is missing to learn to 'float' in the human social environment. There is a clear need to train pediatricians and other social and health workers to have the skills to assess these environmental aspects. The time is perhaps mature. In the editorial of latest issue of an important scientific journal, we read these important sentences: "In primary care settings, the focus on assessing and enhancing caregiver sensitivity in early childhood is not yet a standard of care in general health promotion as is the routine focus on diet, safety, speech and language, cognitive, motor skills, and immunizations. The available data now indicate that assessment of and attention to care giving practices should become a routine part of pediatric primary care"[21]

---

[21] Luby J L, *Editorial: The primacy of parenting*, Child Psychology and Psychiatry, April 2020, 61,4

Chapter 10

Conclusions: What to do?

Need for a moratorium on childhood diagnoses and a return to developmental psychology

The current situation with regard to autism therefore seems to have failed:

the research is bogged down in repetitive and stereotyped declarations of the Authorities of Autism System that exalt the magnificent and progressive fortunes but almost compulsively repeat the mantra of the need for further research to confirm the shining results, etc., etc.;

assistance is based on increasingly bureaucratic and dogmatic programs that risk to ensure the growing interests of groups doing business with the autistic spectrum than to help people who end up in this tunnel;

operators at various levels are 'experts' only in bureaucratic and testing procedures and in the application of training methods that often do not respect people's needs and rights. They no longer have clinical skills and broad assessment skills, but only mechanically and uncritically perform standardized reward/punishment based procedures;

these operators obviously need work and there is therefore a spasmodic search for autistic or presumed autistic children, in nursery schools, in schools. here teachers or educators risk being reduced to advertising consultants for these centers;

with all this, an epidemic of (false) autism spectrum diagnoses is spreading that has now clogged public services with waiting lists of years for interventions such as psychomotricity, speech therapy, etc., however non-specific and palliative;

last but not least, young children and families are thrown into distressing tunnels that disrupt their lives with devastating perspectives at an increasingly early age. The arrogance of some operators is even going so far as to blackmail and threaten to report to the Juvenile Court those families who refuse the proposed interventions.

In all this, 'Science' (a pseudo-science, in reality), called into question by the Health Authorities and the Autistic System to justify partial choices of health policy, is reduced to repetitive slang formulas in which the 'ipse dixit', the consensus of the authorities, prevails in the absence of any real scientific evidence.

We seem to have the elements to raise the alarm of a real health emergency in this field, for the spread of a bad health practice, that almost nobody dares to denounce so far, even if here and there are criticisms but only in the field of insiders.

The public expression of these criticisms and the first signs of denunciation of a now unbearable situation have already provoked opposition reactions from 'stakeholders' in the field. In particular, the first to react to ideas different from those now dominant are certain associations that claim to defend the interests of people declared autistic. They tend to willfully attack the different positions trying to prevent their spread. These people fear the loss of possibilities of assistance for themselves or their relatives. These however - at least so far in Italy, it may be different in other countries - would seem to be fears without reason because assistance to children during development is guaranteed regardless of the diagnosis. Also assistance to people with disabilities and handicaps is guaranteed by law (L 104/92: the so-called Handicap Law, in Italy), regardless of the diagnosis. If there are deficiencies or insufficiencies, it would seem necessary to take action to remedy them in favor of all those concerned and not only of certain categories. The disabled and the families concerned should have everything to gain from the termination of incorrect procedures based on erroneous beliefs and the search for truly meaningful interventions.

Also at the international level there is awareness of the existence of resistance and opposition to possible changes, essentially for two reasons which are:1) the fear of those concerned and their families to lose the interventions and economic aid bureaucratically linked to the diagnosis of autism or autism spectrum. This is especially true in countries with assistance based mainly on private insurance; as was said in a country such as ours, there should not be this danger given the current policy of providing health care to the population regardless or almost regardless of the diagnosis. 2) the concern of health care workers trained exclusively on the current guidelines of intervention for autistic people who would find themselves excluded from the labor market or in the need to broaden their training for new needs.

Then there are the widespread interests of a varied establishment, at the level of universities, research centers, public and private services, ministerial bodies, which in the last decade has reached dominant positions. As is well known, some have even managed to promulgate specific laws on assistance to autism, even with indications of the specific techniques and models to follow, something quite unusual in the medical field and not free from possible suspicions of conflicting interests.

A change in the care of children and neuropsychic developmental difficulties seems therefore necessary and a petition via change.org was launched in August 2019 to draw the attention of the Italian Minister of Health to this situation, and other initiatives followed. (see Appendix 4)

It is appropriate to take note - and first of all to be aware of - the growing criticism of the current model of intervention in the field of autism, the diagnostic criteria used and the epistemological validity of the diagnosis and concept of autism and autism spectrum. As described in Appendix 1, relating to the current debate, internationally recognized scientific authorities in the field of autism also admit, albeit somewhat begrudgingly, the mistakes made and the need to change things.

Therefore, the first thing that seems possible, useful and necessary in our country is a MORATORIUM, i.e. a suspension of the diagnosis of autism and autism spectrum and a shift of the main health objective in this field from the search for the disease to attention to the child's person and his family and all the possible factors at stake. The diagnoses made thus far and the attempt to anticipate it more and more have in fact turned out to be deleterious tools.

Until such time as scientific medical research is re-organized more correctly, addresses errors that have so far affected the results and leads to new proven biological and genetic knowledge, it seems necessary to refocus attention on child development under current social conditions and possible factors that may hinder and facilitate it. In recent years, in fact, the prevalence of attention towards autism has progressively diverted attention away from the most common difficulties of child psychic development, relegating to the sidelines the knowledge known in developmental psychology, with the effect of seriously worsening the care of children and their families.

In practice, it is necessary to overturn the current working methods that follow the notorious 'guidelines' that only look after autistics (or fishing with increasingly narrow 'nets'). Instead of starting from the 'diagnosis' to give the usual repetitive and stereotyped indications the same for everyone, it will be necessary to start from the individual situation of the child and his family to intervene on the critical aspects that may be in focus, medical, psychological or environmental.

It will also be necessary to be well attentive to the effects that the operators' proposals have on families, not to alter their equilibrium except after a conscious discussion and to support the parents in their psychological reactions to the difficulties and interventions in progress. Parents are in fact always fundamental parts in the 'recovery' of their child.

It is important to underline that the objective of the intervention is not merely 'abilitative', i.e. aimed at the acquisition by a child of certain abilities within a certain time, but to facilitate the evolution of the child's personality in all its aspects. The child should not be seen as a series of detached, partial skills and performances, but as a person in its entirety, in its global characteristics as a human being.

Operationally, in my opinion, at the first contact with a situation of evolutionary difficulties, a phase of cognitive observation of the child together with his family should be initiated, which aims to focus on all aspects of the situation, both the possible physical abnormalities of the child (if necessary with medical examinations, EEG, resonance, metabolic, hormonal, genetic, auditory abilities - in addition to a neuro-motor evaluation), as well as the characteristics of his behavior in the family and with strangers and the interactive and communication modalities, care and daily management by the so-called caregivers. It is also essential to have a careful anamnesis, not only medical, but also to take into account the experiences that children and families have lived through, and the possible conditions of environmental isolation and lack of social contact with the repercussions on the mood of the various people and the family climate. This phase, outpatient, intensive enough if possible, or with short hospitalizations if necessary for the distance, should be able to identify possible medical alterations or possible non-optimal ways of care or other environmental needs, to start a subsequent phase of modification of these aspects also with the proposal of experiences useful for psychomotor development.

In these early stages there should be no spasmodic research of the diagnosis, if no specific elements of brain or general abnormalities emerge from the medical examinations, but only use an 'awaiting diagnosis' on the type of ESSENCE proposed in Sweden by C Gillberg almost ten years ago (Appendix 2). The formula could also be *'Neuro-Psychic Developmental Difficulties to Deepen'-DNPDD*, so to say. We stress 'neuro-psychic' to oppose the current 'neuro-developmental' formula, which seems to want to exclude the psychic and relational component from the field of human development.

Obviously, all this can only happen on an enlarged scale if the proposal for a moratorium on autism spectrum diagnosis for children with developmental difficulties is accepted and if the current guidelines in force and the consequent organization of Child Health Services are modified, for a reasonable period of rethinking the whole issue of neuropsychic developmental alterations in young children.

In this way we could begin to help these children and families to free themselves from the 'autism bubble' of which we have spoken and perhaps from the many individual and family 'bubbles' in which they have been imprisoned, so that they can get out into the open air and return to more livable and developmentally friendly living conditions.

Appendix 1

Debate on 'abandoning autism': historical hints of a controversy.

It may be useful to report the essential stages of a debate that has existed for almost a decade at an international level on the usefulness and validity or not of the diagnosis of Autistic Spectrum, of which there is almost no trace in Italy, except for the information that I have tried to give on my site.

As described in various chapters, in recent decades the field of autism has come to configure itself, following the classification of the DSM5 promulgated by the American Psychiatric Association, in a single diagnostic category that collects all developmental disorders previously considered separately. It now remains the only category of 'autism spectrum', divided into three degrees of severity and placed among the so-called 'neurodevelopmental disorders' (neurodevelopmental disorders). This classification has invaded the world almost without resistance, but in the last decade critical positions have begun to appear more or less openly, isolated and silent at first, but which have gradually led the authorities of autism to recognize the difficulties reported and the need for change, at least in research.

A first criticism of the usefulness of the diagnostic categories in use, in the face of too many diagnostic errors and the unreliability of early childhood diagnoses, was in 2010[22] the proposal of C Gillberg, of the University of Gothenburg, Sweden, of the concept of ESSENCE (Early Symptomatic Syndromes Eliciting Neurodevelopmental Clinical Examination). This formula should be used as an all-inclusive generic diagnostic formula in which to group all situations of developmental alteration, from the autistic spectrum to hyperactivity, language disorder, etc., often poorly distinguishable and variable over time, as a waiting diagnosis to be used to avoid too many diagnostic errors. (See Appendix 2)

A second moment was the publication in 2012 in America of the book "Rethinking Autism" by Dr Lynn Waterhouse [23]of the University of New Jersey, USA (see Chapter 5). The book as we have seen systematically and thoroughly examines a quantity of data and research results of the last twenty years on the causes, symptomatology, evolution and treatment of autism. The book as we have seen systematically and thoroughly examines a quantity of data and research results of the last twenty years on the

[22]Gillberg C., *The ESSENCE in child psychiatry: Early Symptomatic Syndromes Eliciting Neurodevelopmental Clinical Examinations,* Res Dev Disabil. Nov-Dec;31(6):1543-51 (2010)
https://www.ncbi.nlm.nih.gov/pubmed/20634041/
[23]Waterhouse L., *Rethinking-Autism* Academic Press, 2012https://www.amazon.com/Rethinking-Autism-Complexity-Waterhouse-2012-09-26/dp/B01FKWOPRG/

causes, symptomatology, evolution and treatment of autism. The conclusion is so much effort and funding has practically failed to find the cause of autism and a reliable treatment. The author goes so far as to state that there is no specific pathology responsible for autism and there is not even an 'autism' in itself, nor a spectrum of related disorders. There are only disparate autistic symptoms which, like fever, are not a disease per se, but the result of different causes. She concludes by making the proposal to radically change the methods, criteria, concepts of research, starting from giving up the diagnosis of autism.

In July 2014 Lynn Waterhouse and Christopher Gillberg reaffirm the need to abandon, dismantle, the concept of autism. Their article is entitled 'Why Autism Must Be Taken Apart'. The abstract reads: "Although more and more evidence is emerging that autism is found in many different brain dysfunctions, researchers have tried to find a single brain dysfunction that would provide neurobiological validity for autism", without success. ... The belief that there is a single brain dysfunction that defines the autism spectrum must be abandoned. Researchers must explore individual variations... "[24].

The proposed new conceptualization, which calls for an extensive search for the relationship between symptoms and possible different brain dysfunctions, renouncing a unifying theory of autism, remains always within an exclusively neurobiological vision, but at least it does justice to sensational conceptual and methodological errors that

---

[24]Waterhouse L., Gillberg C., *Why Autism Must be Taken Apart* Autism Dev Disord. ul;44(7):1788-92, (2014)

are recognized at this point as a serious obstacle to the progress of knowledge in the field.

Another critical voice in the current diagnosis of Autism/Autism Spectrum is Eric London, of the New York State Institute for Basic Research in Developmental Disabilities, Albany, NY, USA, who already wrote an article in 2014 with the unequivocal title: "Categorical diagnosis: a fatal flaw for autism research?" [25].

In a 'conversation' in 2105 [26] the author clarifies various critical aspects of the diagnosis of autism. "Such a diagnosis has falsely given the idea that we know the issue well. Paradoxically, this discourages further investigation and reduces the information a doctor may have available". On the other hand, he says, "it is a sad fact to see this, but orthodoxies die slowly, and science - which should be guided by evidence - tends to be as conservative as anything else". London therefore recommends setting aside autism spectrum diagnosis and using 'Brain Developmental Disorder' as a global diagnosis instead of dealing with symptoms in relation to brain development. Attention should be focused on the different symptoms and clinical pictures to analyze them in depth. He also states that DSM5 has not been useful in clarifying the field of developmental disorders and recalls that the National Institute of Mental Health, the main U.S. mental health agency, in 2013 proposed an alternative to DSM with the RDoC system, 'Re-

[25]London, E., *Categorical diagnosis: a fatal flaw for autism research?*, Trends Neurosci. 2014 Dec;37(12):683-6. doi: 10.1016/j.tins.2014.10.003. Epub 2014 Nov 14.

[26]https://www.spectrumnews.org/opinion/questions-for-ric-london-alternati...

search Domain Criteria', to focus attention on the functions at stake, rather than on categorical diagnoses.

In April 2015 a geneticist, Thomas Bourgeron, of the Human Genetics and Cognitive Functions Unit, Institute Pasteur, Paris, France, takes a so to speak intermediate position in a Lecture on 'The genetics and neurobiology of ESSENCE'. On the one hand it seems to accept Waterhouse and Gillberg's invitation to abandon autism ("As suggested by Waterhouse and Gillberg it might be better to abandon the belief that there is a single brain dysfunction at the basis of the Autistic Spectrum") and on the other hand it advocates further biological research on ESSENCE, confirming the idea of this category as a new all-encompassing diagnosis of the disease that would affect 10% of children (and by the numbers it might attract even more research funding).

Later, in December 2016, a new article entitled Autistic Spectrum Disorder Validity (ASD Validity)[27] appeared, in which Waterhouse , London, and Gillberg join their efforts to once again reaffirm that the diagnosis of Autistic Spectrum Disorder(ASD) is devoid of biological and logical-scientific validity. The authors affirm the need to abandon this concept, the diagnosis of ASD and the related criteria, both in the field of research and in the field of the clinic. They add that there is likely to be strong resistance to this major change, due to the magnitude of the interests at stake.

---

[27]Waterhouse L, London E & Gillberg,C, *Autism Spectrum Disorder Validity,* Review Journal of Autism and Developmental Disorders, Volume 3, Issue 4, pp 302–329 (2016)

In January 2107 the editorial of Autism research - official journal of the International Society for Autism Research - entitled "Time to give up on Autism Spectrum Disorder? " [28] finally takes a position on the subject. Bourgeron admits the existence of difficulties and problems deriving from the terminology and concepts used so far, unduly unifying a situation that instead presents a great heterogeneity, but rejects the need to change everything.

The impression is that this is an ex officio defense by the official authorities, so to speak, of the Autistic Spectrum. The arguments try to reject the criticism and refuse to give up the concepts and tools used so far, but recognize the existence of problems to be better addressed, first of all the great heterogeneity of the cases collected under the unifying umbrella of the Autism Spectrum Disorders, and similarly the presence of autistic-like 'symptoms' in different situations.

On 2 March 2017 C. Gillberg in his blog at the University Centre in Gothenburg, which bears his name, returns to the subject with a significant title, "No more religious faith in ADI/ADOS" . In this post he informs about the ongoing debate on the validity of the autistic spectrum and stigmatizes the now widespread use of making diagnoses only with tests. He comments that many people are concerned that the changes envisaged will lead to the loss of services for people with problems who currently have the diagnostic label of Autism. Gillberg says he is an advo-

---

[28]Muller R A, Amaral DG., *Editorial: Time to give up on Autism Spectrum Disorder?*, Autism Res. Jan;10(1):10-14, (2017)
https://www.ncbi.nlm.nih.gov/pubmed/28130875/

cate for the decomposition of autism in research, while he believes it is still premature to do so in clinical activity. There is a need, according to him, to find concepts that better capture the clinical manifestations and to modify the specialized services for individuals with 'autism'. He sees the training of staff for new needs as a serious problem. Currently, in his opinion (which I think is very sharable), operators involved in autism have relatively little experience in the field of the different neuro-evolutionary disorders including ESSENCE and seem to believe almost blindly in the algorithms of ADOS or ADI as 'specific tools for autism', used 'as magic solutions - abracadabra - with no more room for a global expert clinical evaluation'.

Later, in July 2017, in *Autism Research* [29], Lynn Waterhouse, Eric London, Christopher Gillberg, write a letter to the publisher entitled "The ASD diagnosis has blocked the discovery of valid biological variation in neurodevelopmental social impairment" and try again to draw the attention of the scientific community to the serious problems of autism research arising from the prevailing diagnostic settings.

In response, another letter is published in the same issue, "Abandoning ASD? A response to Waterhouse, London, and Gillberg" by Ralph-Axel Müller, co-editor of Autism Research, who quite disdainfully rejects the idea of abandoning the concept of autism, and says that researchers

---

[29]Waterhouse L, London E, Gillberg C, *The ASD diagnosis has blocked the discovery of valid biological variation in neurodevelopmental social impairment* , Autism Research Volume 10, Issue 7, *2017*https://onlinelibrary.wiley.com/doi/abs/10.1002/aur.1832/

are aware that the diagnosis of Autistic Spectrum includes many different types of neurobiological disorders, but that it is better, instead of abandoning autism, to improve research methods...

On January 7, 2019 on Molecular Psychiatry [30]appears an article by Michael V Lombardo, Meng-Chuan Lai & Simon Baron-Cohen - the latter a well-known name in the field - who admit that research on autism so far has not taken into account the great heterogeneity of cases and that this has produced failed data. They therefore claim that it is 'imperative' to change course. It seems like an attempt to run for cover, 'trying to save goat and cabbage', hiding behind methodological criteria.

In short, at an international level there seems to be a crescendo of criticism that if nothing else has led to the awareness of evident critical aspects in the dominant view of autism.

What about Italy? Maybe something's moving, even if it's out of the spotlight.

EmidioTribulato, of the Centro Studi Logos of Messina, in his book 'Autism and Free Self-Managed Play' [31]of 2013 describes a vision of autism that criticizes the exclusively bio-genetic vulgate of autism and gives space to the emotional and relational aspects. It describes and proposes a mode of intervention with the child based on 'self-managed free play' as an essential tool to free the autistic child from

[30]Lombardo V., Meng-Chuan Lai & Baron-Cohen S, *Big data approaches to decomposing heterogeneity across the autism spectrum* Molecular psychiatry 7 gennaio 2019 https://www.nature.com/articles/s41380-018-0321-0/
[31]Tribulato E., *Autismo e gioco libero autogestito,* Franco Angeli editore,(2013)

the constraints often unconsciously imposed by adults. In the book's conclusions, it debunks many false beliefs about 'autistic children' and ends up saying that 'they are not children to be educated but to be freed' from the suffering and constraints that block their development and life.

Michele Zappella[32] denies the exponential growth in the diagnosis of Autistic Spectrum and explains this increase as an error due essentially to 3 factors: - 1) the disappearance of the distinction between autism and other situations of developmental difficulty that were previously evaluated in the necessary differential diagnosis; - 2) the uncritical use of the tests in vogue, which cause too many false positives; and 3) the use of the criteria established with the DSM5. In this regard it states that the countries in which the autistic spectrum epidemic occurs are all DSM5-compliant. A comparison with the epidemiological data of countries that instead refer to the ICD10, the WHO's classification of diseases, including France, China and others, shows that in these countries the diagnoses have not had the same surge. Zappella also stresses the importance of the way in which the assessment is carried out, criticising the objective mechanical methods in vogue today.

Flavia Capozzi in 2017, in an extensive article published on the web page of the Italian Psychoanalytical Society [33], makes a careful criticism of the changes in the field of autism, at the level of definition, diagnostic criteria,

---

[32]Zappella, M *Difficoltà diagnostiche in bambini con disturbi del neurosviluppo* Autismo e Disturbi dello Sviluppo',17(2):169-183 (2019)

[33]Capozzi, F., *Autismo e la società 4.0: la psicoanalisi ha ancora diritto di parola?,* spiweb approfondimenti dossier, 12 ottobre 2017

https://www.spiweb.it/dossier/umani-robot-una-relazione-pericolosa-ottob.../

research on causes and treatment. The author believes that the new definition of DSM5 - and in Italy the guidelines of the Istituto Superiore di Sanità of 2011 - define autism in a too reductive way and underlines how it is probably causing both the abnormal increase in the number of diagnoses and the orientation of families and health policy towards inappropriate and undifferentiated therapeutic choices. It also points out that research over the last 20 years has focused mainly on investigating the role of genetic factors with less satisfactory results than promised and has had little interest in the complex etiological role played by psycho-socio-environmental factors and in particular the interaction between genes, environment and society.

As for the treatment, the author notes that at the moment there is a lack of reliable research on the treatment of autism and comments that we are witnessing a homologation and simplification of methods that is proceeding towards a unique, intensive educational model, with more training than empowering intentions. He points out that this perspective, which sees the child with autism "no longer as a psychotic but as a disabled person" (quoting S.Lebovici, French psychoanalyst of the last century), leaves families without psychological assistance. Indeed, parents, after receiving such a dramatic diagnosis for the future of their children, are often left alone without a guide, a psychological support that accompanies them through a difficult process of growth and helps them to choose the most suitable course of treatment.

On the whole, therefore, there are also in Italy several critical positions of the current situation, but isolated and not very visible. Apparently, the echo of the debate that directly questions the diagnosis and the very concept of autism has not yet arrived.

For my part, for years I have been writing on my website about existing things, for my 23 visitors. In September 2019 the journal of the Medici Order of Florence, Toscana Medica, hosted an article of mine entitled "Is the autism bubble about to burst?"[34] in which I informed my colleagues about the state of the debate we are talking about here, which was followed in the same issue by a response article that represented the official position. Then there was my petition via change.org (Appendix 4) with a subsequent press conference in Pistoia, Tuscany, that had a fair repercussion in the local news.

---

[34] Benedetti G, Sta per scoppiare la bolla dell'autismo?, Toscana Medica, 8/2019

Appendix 2

From the Autistic Spectrum to ESSENCE

This section concerns some proposals to change the diagnosis system in use today for children with neuropsychic developmental difficulties, based on the DSM5. These proposals have been made at an international level in recent years due to the growing criticism of these diagnoses, as illustrated elsewhere in the book.

As already mentioned, supporters of the theory of autism as a neurobiological disorder were confronted with the fact that children who initially fell within the classifying criteria of the Autistic Spectrum, in the following years could present so different characteristics that they had to change their diagnosis, especially in ADHD, language disorders, Tourette's syndrome, and others. Not to talk about how many were "coming out from the diagnosis" which, therefore, turned out to be wrong (because, by definition, autism is incurable), result of diagnostic errors from wrong tests or from careless operators in whose hands the tests for autism have become dangerous weapons. As we have seen, it had to be concluded that the criteria to diagnose autism were in reality not specific and reliable enough and that therefore too many fish-children besides the presumed autistic ones remained imprisoned in the nets because of the too thick meshes. While in reality small fish are protected by clear fishing regulations, this is not the case for children. This is perhaps something akin to what happened in the early twentieth century when, in order to protect children, animal protection regulations had to be invoked, at least in England.

The ESSENCE was, I believe, the first proposal to put aside the diagnoses commonly used in young children and replace them with different ways of considering them. This proposal was made in 2010 by the Swedish child psychiatrist Cristopher Gillberg, considered one of the most authoritative scholars in the field of autism and child psychiatry in general, certainly the most prolific of scientific publications on the subject. Gillberg coined, in a 2010 article [35], the acronym of ESSENCE, which means 'Early Symptomatic Syndromes Eliciting Neurodevelopmental Clinical Examinations'.

The new 'box' with this name in its intentions should therefore collect situations with difficulties such as: "(a) general development, (b) communication and language, (c) social interaction, (d) motor coordination, (e) attention/hearing, (f) activity, (g) behavior, (h) mood and (i) sleep. These up to now are classified according to DSM5 in

---

[35] Gillberg C., The ESSENCE in child psychiatry: Early Symptomatic Syndromes Eliciting Neurodevelopmental Clinical Examinations. Res Dev Disabil. 2010 Nov-Dec;31(6):1543-51
https://www.ncbi.nlm.nih.gov/pubmed/20634041

categorical diagnoses, i.e. of specific diseases: ADHD, Autistic Spectrum, Coordination Developmental Disorder, Intellectual Developmental Disorder, 'specific' language disorders, Tourette's syndrome, early bipolar disorders, genetic behavioral syndromes, and a variety of neurological and convulsive disorders that present with behavioral and cognitive alterations at an early age". Gillberg stresses that Essence is not a diagnosis in itself but "a conceptual tool that allows a step forward, alerting clinicians and researchers to the wide variety of problems manifested by children, adolescents and adults with all kinds of neurodevelopmental problems of early origin".

In 2013, the concept was re-proposed again and seems to have entered into use in various parts of the world. In Italy, too, a few conferences have been held to present the concept, but little more, at least so far. In spring 2018 an international conference was held in Gothenburg to collect the results of the first years of use of this concept. ESSENCE should be in practice a kind of all-inclusive 'waiting diagnosis', an 'umbrella' diagnosis that brings together all young children who end up with specialists for problems inherent to their neuropsychic development. Prolonged clinical observation is considered necessary in order to clarify their clinical picture and to avoid the aforementioned diagnostic errors with their consequences of wrong interventions and unjustified suffering. It is not a renunciation of diagnosis, but a form of caution in the face of too many mistakes made. The emphasis placed so far on the precocity of the diagnosis is instead shifted to the correctness and completeness of the knowledge of the different situations.

A further consequence of the concept of ESSENCE, declared by the promoters, is that it is not appropriate, according to them, to create centers highly specialized in specific diseases, such as the specific centers for the diagnosis of autism that have also spread in Italy, because of the excess of false positives that this would inevitably create. But it is much more appropriate to create centers for the evaluation of neuropsychic development able to deepen the examination of the different situations that arise and to follow the development of children with the appropriate interventions in individual cases.

In reality, that of the ESSENCE seems to be an attempt to solve one of the most difficult problems that the researchers of autism were facing, as written in the text itself: that of the ill-famed 'comorbidity' and confusion between the various disorders indicated, which are difficult to separate, which overlap one another and which can fall under one or the other diagnosis over time, creating precisely the confusion that we are witnessing today. As mentioned above, we go as far as the case of children 'out of diagnosis' of diseases that are considered genetically determined and healless.

Gillberg should be credited with having perceived the contradictions in the construction of autism as early as 10 years ago, perhaps first, and with having tried to run for cover. It is also a sign that the field of research on autism was flaking a bit in the face of the increasingly serious and unresolved problems that the concepts of autism and the autistic spectrum had created.

A few years later, in 2014, another proposal was made in New York to radically change the diagnostic system in place. Erik London, as we have seen also in Appendix 1 of the 'debate', proposed a more 'neurological' umbrella diagnosis, to collect all the cases of children so far variously diagnosed, that of 'brain developmental disorder'. London regretted in an interview[36] that there were too few brains of people with neuro-developmental disorders to analyze and considered this one of the main reasons for the failure of autism research. He proposed to try to establish a brain bank for the future that researchers could draw on for various anatomical, histological and biological studies.

It must be said that even C Gillberg and his group and L Waterhouse herself remain in the field of neurological research, in the conception that neuro-developmental disorders have only neurobiological causes. Even if they do not dare, probably because of their purely neurological training, to go beyond the limits of a vision that excludes half of the sky, so to speak, that is all the possible non-neurological factors of developmental alteration, they must be given the merit of having denounced the critical aspects of the autism system and of insisting on their denunciation for several years, despite the opposition of the majority of the autism research and care system.

---

[36]Interview with dr Eric London https://autismsciencefoundation.org/what-is-autism/autism-science/interviews-with-scientists/dr-eric-london-new-york-state-institute-for-basic-research-in-developmental-disabilities/

We are therefore faced with more proposals to change everything in the diagnosis of neuropsychic disorders in young children. If Gillberg's proposal were to make its way, the positive thing is that instead of the terrifying sound of Autistic Spectrum, parents will find in their ears the somewhat more anonymous one of 'ESSENCE', which will make the French think first about petrol, since that is what it is called in French. But the other side of the coin will be that the statistics on neuropsychic disorders of childhood will go from 1 to 38 (clearly a figure distorted by the unreliable criteria currently in vogue) as now for the autistic spectrum, to 1 to 10 (!) for ESSENCE disorders, and children and families will be increasingly medicalized, psychologized and psychiatricized...

Appendix 3

The so-called institutional autism

An important aspect to remember in the debate on autism is that of so-called 'institutional autism'. The term was used by Michael Rutter and others [37] in the 1990s and 2000s to refer to cases of children from orphanages in Romania and other Eastern European countries being adopted at an early age by Western families with symptoms that overlapped those of autistic children tout court. These children after varying periods of time often lost their autistic characteristics to resume normal or almost normal development. It was considered a 'natural experiment' on the effect of environmental conditions on psychic development. Even in my experience over the years I have followed similar situations. The characteristics of these children were

---

[37] Rutter M. et al, *Longitudinal Studies Using a "Natural Experiment" Design: The Case of Adoptees From Romanian Institution*s,Journal of the American Academy of Child & Adolescent PsychiatryVolume 51, Issue 8, August 2012, Pages 762-770   Among other things, the study shows that social deprivation is associated with a marked increase in mental disorders and that if the stay in the institution was longer than six months there was also a reduction in the cranial circumference, not due to malnutrition.

easily attributed to the conditions in which they had lived for more or less long periods, in unorganized institutions to provide them with assistance useful for their mental development but only for physical survival. If the adoption took place within a certain age and if the period of hospitalization was not too long, the children's conditions improved quite quickly. The symptoms of developmental retardation and a tendency to isolation and avoid social contact were in many cases quite comparable to those of typical autism cases.

On the other hand, in the years of the Second World War and soon afterwards, many psychological studies were carried out on children abandoned because of the war and hospitalized in British institutions. These studies had denounced the serious repercussions of those living conditions on the development and mental health of children. Anna Freud [38], René Spitz and others described typical pictures of arrested mental development even with physical impairment (described with terms such as 'Hospitalism' and 'anaclitic depression') and brought impetus to the theories that signaled the importance of emotional and affective environmental conditions for the development of children. Also in England, in the following years, a movement developed that led to the organization of pediatric hospitals in a new way, allowing the presence of a family member next to the hospitalized child, something that did not happen before and that in Italy began to spread only in the late seventies. In Italy, again from the seventies onwards, a move-

---

[38] Burlingham, D., & Freud, A. (1944). Infants without families. Allen & Unwin.

ment developed that led to the closure of both psychiatric hospitals and institutions for handicapped children. At that time, in the first years of my professional activity I was able to verify such situations, working for periods both in institutions of chronic hospitalization and in day care centers. Comparing this with today, I can see the different evolution of children with genetic anomalies, who at that time often ended up in institutions and now live in families. A good part of children with Down's syndrome (Trisomy 21) at that time had a serious picture of mental retardation and autistic manifestations, with isolation, absence of language, stereotypes, etc., while today people with these diseases, which remain unchanged in frequency, almost never show such serious clinical pictures.

All these elements show the importance of the environmental conditions of emotional and affective care, of the experiences that a child may or may not have, for his or her development, and they all show the importance of more careful research and study of developmental psychology and the factors involved, a subject that has remained on the margins in these decades of research dedicated mainly to biological factors.

Appendix 4

A Petition to the Italian Minister of Health, via change.org

In August 2019, in the face of the immobility of the Italian situation (in the field of autism and in the face of the umpteenth situations of malpractice, you could say, bring me back to families caught in the infamous networks of autism, I tried to move the environment a little bit out of the limits of my website with an online petition via change.org addressed to the Minister of Health. The petition in mid-September was forwarded via email to the minister's secretariat, who had just taken office. I had the pleasant surprise of being called back the same day by a physician-functionary of the Minister's secretariat who assured me of his interest and attention to the subject and my comments. It is a pity that I did not have any other news afterwards. The current coronavirus pandemic has made more urgent needs prevail, but the problems described do not cease to exist.

Here is the text, which can be viewed by adding your signature on the change.org page [39]

I am a 70 year old child neuropsychiatrist with over 45 years of experience in the field. I continue to see families and children with evolutionary difficulties of various nature and degree that are overwhelmed in the vicious mechanism that has been created between nurseries, kindergartens, pediatricians and specialized services to catch more and more cases of 'autistic spectrum' to be initiated to the usual interventions, the same for all different situations, in the public and especially in the private sector, since now the waiting lists are increasingly long.

Children with difficulties that are often transitory or in any case variously understandable and different from each other are caught in the 'net' of the system indicated above, which catches increasingly smaller 'fish' often disrupting their lives and those of their families. This is due to serious diagnostic and evaluation errors made more frequent than ever by the current approach, based on quantitative mechanical tests and evaluations that do not take into account the quality of environmental situations and experiences.

It is probable that at the basis of the evolution we are witnessing, rather dismayed, are the changes in the clinic and in the organization of the diagnostic and care services that are represented in the notorious Guidelines for Autism, issued at the official level by the health authorities. I believe that these guidelines are deeply flawed and should be taken into consideration in order to change them greatly.

---

[39] Change org, Petition http://chng.it/Zc6bChdLQj/

In addition, from various parts of the world, from America, to England, to Sweden, voices are raised against the current view of autism and the autism spectrum, proposing to reconsider everything, in the face of the failure of research on autism, which has not been able to find causes or reliable remedies. It is proposed to renounce the very term of autism, and its diagnosis, as conceptually and clinically wrong. It was proposed, particularly in young children who come to the observation, to no longer make specific diagnoses but to consider them as a group (ESSENCE, C. Gillberg) to be followed and observed in depth, at wide range, in a differentiated and individualized way, in order to find specific factors and individual remedies case by case.

Since in 2015 the Parliament made a law regulating interventions in the field of autism (I do not know if there are other 'diseases' that have had this honor...), delegating to the health authorities the task of dealing with it, it is likely that by now the issue will have to move from politics, with all the complications that follow. In 2016, a National Autism Observatory was set up by the Ministry of Health, which expresses the official position that seems to us so profoundly wrong.

I believe that the Ministry of Health should not remain insensitive to the cry of pain of so many devastated families that I am trying to convey with this appeal, and should start rethinking the whole situation, with the necessary transparency that is not there today and risks covering organized interests in conflict with the interests of public health. (end of the text of the petition)

Appendix 5

Definitions of autism. Comparison of questions/answers

Here is a representative definition of the current vulgate of autism as a 'neurodevelopmental disorder' due to 'definitely neurobiological' causes, which can be found on an internet page of an Italian pediatrics magazine [40]. We take it as an example for its simplicity and clarity, and because it is addressed to the parents of small children, the main users and injured parties of the situation:

"Autism is a set of alterations in brain development, variable from one subject to another, which involve a compromise of social skills and language, as well as various behavioural disorders".

In our view, the above definition is worthless because it hypothesizes pathogenic causes and mechanisms ("*set of alterations in brain development,*") that have never been found - without specifying which alterations, by the

---

[40]Calia V., *autismo e disturbi dello spettro autistico,* Un pediatra come amico, 4/11/2019 *https://www.uppa.it/medicina/malattie-e-disturbi/autismo-disturbi-dello-spettro-autistico/*

way. Then the author will contradict himself by saying (in subsequent answers) that the causes are unknown.

Lacking a valid definition, there is little progress in epidemiology and science, but there is a lot of smoke and confusion, which is perhaps what many people are looking for, to prevent them from seeing things well. The lack of a valid definition is actually the fundamental error that has made the search for causes and remedies of such an indefinite object fail. In my opinion it is more correct to say, using the same words in another sequence:

"There are people with compromised social skills and language as well as with various behavioral disorders, varying from one subject to another, the causes of which are unknown. These people are called 'autistic'".

The diagnostic category corresponding to the symptoms has been called 'autistic disorder' or recently 'autistic spectrum disorder'. In itself it is an indefinite (spectral) phantom entity and a tautological definition: 'autism is what produces autistic symptoms'. Then follow on the same page a series of questions and answers. Let's summarize the original answers below and follow with our own.

1 *What is autism?* It is said that it is not a disorder defined with certainty but rather a set of disorders for which today we use the term 'autistic spectrum'. It is admitted that these disorders are variable from one subject to another and therefore each one is a case in itself.

For my part I would say that it is a term to indicate a behavior closed in itself. No real scientific evidence has been found so far that it is also a disease that causes the so-called autistic symptoms. The causes of such behavior can

110

be the most diverse, some known (genetic or metabolic or inflammatory brain diseases) and others not.

2 *What are the symptoms of autism*? The official answer is a list of difficulties visible since early childhood, "more or less present and accentuated", ranging from those of language, both spoken and non-verbal; and then of sociality; imagination, with narrow interests and rigid and repetitive behavior; emotionality; the ability to self-regulate and self-control. It is pointed out that some subjects can have very high cognitive abilities and also musical and mathematical abilities (and here the thought obviously goes to Mozart and Einstein, enlisted in the ranks of autistic geniuses) while others have reduced cognitive abilities. It is emphasized that without treatment the symptoms will get worse... The vagueness and indeterminacy is such that every parent or almost every parent fears to see his or her child there.

My answer is that in general autistic symptoms are considered as not caring and not having interest and curiosity in getting in touch with people. The development of language and symbolic, cognitive and social skills can have various difficulties. However, they are not 'specific' symptoms but aspects common to various situations.

3 *What does 'high functioning autism' mean*? The official answer is caution: there is a wide diversity of abilities and difficulties, the presence of good language and good intelligence (even extraordinary in some, sic!) distinguishes high functioning autism from low functioning autism.

I would say that it is a way to distinguish people with autistic behavior with or without mental retardation. The "high functioning" is considered typical of Asperger's syndrome; the statements that Mozart and Einstein were like that maybe contributes to entice some people who prefer to define themselves as affected by this syndrome.

4 *How frequent is autism*? And here it says that they tend to be higher and higher, 1 to 88 at the moment, reports the site. The explanation given for the almost exponential increase in cases, is the greater ability of doctors to make this diagnosis thanks to modern techniques.

In reality it is difficult to talk about the frequency, because the diagnostic criteria have changed over time and now include the most different situations. Today they are called 'autistic' children who once would not have been defined in this way. A rigorous epidemiological method cannot put together different things and think of providing serious answers. As a result, statistics are lost in this maze.

5 *What are the causes of autism*? They admit that the answer is unknown, contradicting the very definition given before. But then they state that it is known that there is an important hereditary component (although there is no comprehensive evidence), and that there is the hypothesis that there are anomalies in the connections between nerve cells that make the brain's abilities "rigid". It states that a basic structure of neuronal networks formed in embryonic life is damaged in autistic subjects, due to possible genetic and congenital prenatal factors, not better defined. The last pearl is that there is no evidence of the influence of exter-

nal environmental, neither physical, nor psychic factors resulting from interaction with parents.

For my part, paraphrasing L Wittgenstein, I would just say that not knowing what is meant by this word cannot even know the causes and it would be better to keep silent. Actually 'science' has not dealt with the relational environmental aspects, so it is a good game to proclaim that there is no evidence of these aspects. In reality, there is no evidence of anything, neither for nor against, one is groping in the dark. That's what they don't want to admit.

6 *What is the future of an autistic child*? Going on, the answer is that the child will never be able to get rid of the "autistic quality" of his incurable condition, and that if no action is taken he can be condemned to a serious disability and exclusion from autonomous social life.

I wonder which parent will not immediately rush to 'cure' his child at the slightest sign.. : my answer is similar to the one above: not knowing what it is, one cannot predict its evolution.

7 *At what age can one diagnose autism*? Here it is said that one could have some suspicion from the first year if there is not a good "visual hook" and in general it is possible to do it within the first two years, in particular if there is a delay in language etc. Fortunately, it warns against possible misdiagnosis.

I'd say there's a lot of propaganda in this regard to anticipate diagnoses. In fact, at the international level, it is proposed not to make any more diagnoses of autism in young children, but only to make a waiting diagnosis, because these diagnoses have proved to be unreliable.

8 *Screening tests for autism.* It is said that, since an early diagnosis is fundamental to start a therapeutic and rehabilitative path, it is important to do screening tests, such as the CHAT (Checklist for Autism in Toddlers) questionnaire with its variants M-CHAT* (Modified chat) and Q-CHAT (Quantitative chat), which allows suspicious cases to be identified and kept under observation.

In fact, screening is under indictment in many areas of medicine because it perhaps produces more harm than good. In our case they are a serious problem because they often induce pediatricians to send a large number of children to autism specialists, without investigating possible other causes of possible delays or abnormalities, thus creating and spreading unjustified panic and distress.

9 *How to diagnose autism?* It is specified that the diagnosis is "clinical" (i.e. there are no blood tests or instrumental tests that can confirm it) and that it is based exclusively on observation of the child or, rather, on the use of internationally recognized tests, such as ADOS-2 (Autism Diagnostic Observation Schedule-2nd Edition), based on observation of the child, and ADI-R (Autism Diagnostic Interview-Revised), based on questions to parents.

In fact, the tendency is now almost everywhere to use only the tests without evaluating the child's situation clinically. This fact is probably responsible for the (false) diagnosis epidemic that we are seeing today. These tests are actually simple measurements of certain behaviors, which in themselves mean nothing. The spread, via the internet and other media, of the knowledge of 'symptoms' (do not look, do not answer, do not say hello, do not indicate,

114

etc., which in reality are also present in many children without problems, as well as the so-called 'stereotypes') is dangerous because it is deforming the attitude of many parents towards their child, from the first months of life.

10 *Brief history of the treatment of autism.* We read that the first attempts to treat autism date back to the 50s of the last century, with the use of intensive and prolonged psychotherapies. Then the psychoanalyst Bruno Bettelheim and his book 'The Empty Fortress' are mentioned, and the concept of "refrigerated mother" and the hypothesis of "coldness" of parents as the cause of autism with the consequent therapeutic proposal to remove autistic children from their families. Other therapies that spread in the last decades of the last century are also mentioned. The "holding therapy" (advocated in Italy by M Zappella) consisted in close physical contact with the autistic child; the Doman method, instead, proposed an intense sensory stimulation; the TEACCH method (acronym of Treatment and Education of Autistic and Communication Handicapped Children), involves the parents themselves in an intense program of teaching, helping them to interact effectively with their children. Then there is a separate chapter on the ABA Method (Applied Behavioral Analysis), which is intended - it is said - to "teach" something to autistic children, who would be 'open to change', provided they are offered an appropriate approach. It is said that the treatment, to be effective, must be intensive: about 20/25 hours a week for 12 months a year, taking place in different contexts of life,

therapeutic centre, family and school, and starting as early as possible.

What can I say? The information is quite accurate historically but perhaps biased, so to speak. History is written by the winners, as we know, and so far the biological behaviorist tendency has won. There is no mention of methods, Denver, DIR, of a less behaviorist and more interpersonal approach. There is in fact no reliable data on the effectiveness of the different treatments, also because the reports can often be biased by conflicts of interest. About Bettelheim, and psychoanalysis in general, an unprecedented attack was concentrated, which was perhaps the cause of his suicide and will make it taboo for many years to study the influences of the environment on children's development. As we saw perhaps 'the times they are a-changin'.

11 *How to choose an effective treatment for autism*? Various therapeutic proposals are mentioned (ABA, Denver, DAN, psychomotricity, speech therapy, facilitated communication, pet therapy, hyperbaric oxygen, PECS, cranio-sacral massage, vitamin B6, mindfulness, water therapy, homeopathy...) and the guidelines of the health authorities would seem to favor the ABA method and, in any case, behaviorist methods.

I dare say that the field has lent itself and lends itself to the most deceptive and fraudulent raids of swindlers and profiteers. On the other hand, if the validity of the concept and diagnosis of autism and autism spectrum is questioned, the whole Cathedral of the Autism System can collapse, with its diagnostic and therapeutic methods so well

116

propagated. It is better to be cautious and not trust and instead try to better understand the child's difficulties on a case-by-case basis, without blindly relying on anyone.

12 *Asperger's Syndrome*. According to the author, Hans Asperger was one of the discoverers of childhood autism and he described a variant that was called with his name. It is - as it is reported - a form of high functioning autism that has some of the typical characteristics of autism spectrum disorders (difficulties in language, verbal and non-verbal communication and empathy), but without compromising intelligence.

Here the historical news must be corrected and integrated. Some decades ago it was proposed to call people with autistic behavior and normal levels of intelligence by the name of the Austrian doctor. He had called them 'autistic psychopaths' in the 1940s. Recent research [41][42] has revealed that during the occupation of Vienna by the Nazis, he appears to have compromised with eugenic programs to eliminate mentally handicapped people. It may now be embarrassing perhaps to identify people with the name of this doctor, and the syndrome with his name has been deleted from the classifications. I am a little puzzled by the number of successful people who recently claim to be suffering from Asperger's disease. It seems to me a phenomenon that has psychological and cultural roots to be better understood in group and social psychology.

---

[41] Herwing Czech, *Hans Asperger, National Socialism, and "race hygiene" in Nazi-era Vienna-Molecular Autism* volume 9, 29 (2018)

[42] Edith Sheffer- *Asperger's Children: The Origins of Autism in Nazi Vienna* - New York: W.W. Norton & Company, (2018)

13 Autism in history (books, cinema, TV and current affairs). Here the author inserts a list of events and manifestations in which autism is the protagonist, citing among other things films, novels, television series and characters such as Mozart, Michelangelo, Newton, Hitchcock and the latest Greta Thumberg. Interested people can go at the source.

It is undoubtedly a very popular subject, and this perhaps explains the great interests at stake.

Appendix 6

Case Study – The little Dick

Re-reading and re-examination of Melanie Klein's famous 1930 article, "The Importance of Symbol-Formation in the Development of the Ego", on a child considered "typically autistic" in retrospect [43]

After my ideas on autism changed in recent years I went to review many of the classic authors of autism and returned to read Melanie Klein's Dick case. I approach it here in the way I would examine a case in a remote consultation, as I have done many times in the last decade, with the new possibilities provided by the web. In this case the distance is also temporal, but otherwise the case lends itself well, it seems to me, to my evaluation methods.

The case of little Dick described in 1930 by Melanie Klein is very famous in the psychoanalytic environment

[43]Klein, M (1930). *The Importance of Symbol-Formation in the Development of the Ego. Int. J. Psycho-Anal.*, 11:24-39 . Republished in 'Contributions to Psychoanalysis', 1921-1945. By Melanie Klein. London: Hogarth Press, 1948. Re-use license N 4773090776859 Cambridge University Press Feb 20, 2020

also because it has been retrospectively recognized as a case of *ante litteram* autism (since psychiatrist Leo Kanner will propose his new diagnosis only 13 years later). It has therefore long attracted the attention of many specialists, including the French psychoanalyst Jacques Lacan and the English psychotherapist Frances Tustin, who was particularly dedicated in her life to autism. We will return to this briefly at the end.

In the text of Klein's article a first part describing the situation of the child is followed by a part that provides us with various anamnesis information. However, nothing is said about the pregnancy, the birth and the condition of the child at birth, and little about the educational and care modalities. However, certain characteristics regarding the environment and the attitude of family members are reported. The author then describes in more detail the first sessions and then the progress of the six months of analysis made with the little patient. Then follows a discussion of the diagnosis of childhood schizophrenia that had been put to the child. M Klein basically agreed, although she raised some significant and very interesting reservations. Finally, in the final part there is a fine-tuning and a summary of the author's theories on child development at that time.

Klein's paper contains many descriptive clinical elements that make the case and its therapy still very interesting to read today. However, it is placed by Klein at the service of her aim to demonstrate her theories of child development and her psychoanalytic technique. Therefore the clinical elements are preceded and followed by the theoretical parts and in addition are interspersed and mixed with

120

theoretical and explanatory comments that often interrupt the reading, weighing it down and perhaps disturbing the understanding of the case.

I have therefore isolated the descriptive part of the text excluding all the theoretical and explanatory elements, in order to read it without interruption. I also reorganized the various information available in a sequence that reflects my way of organizing the anamnestic data.

The result is the text below (in italics the extracts of Klein's almost literal text, reorganized and deprived of the theoretical explanatory cues).

Clinical picture

(Dick is) *a 4 year old child but with a level of linguistic and intellectual development of about 15-18 months, almost devoid of emotional relationship with his environment and ability to adapt to reality. Dick was almost devoid of affectivity and indifferent to the presence or absence of his mother or nanny. From the earliest times he had only rarely shown signs of discomfort and to a low degree.*

With one exception, he had almost no interest, no play, no contact with his environment. For the most part, she simply put together sounds in a meaningless way and repeated certain noises over and over again.

When he spoke, he used his poor vocabulary incorrectly. But that wasn't the only reason why it wasn't understandable: he had no desire to be. Dick was opposed to his mother, often doing just the opposite of what she expected of him. For example, if she could get him to repeat words, he would often cripple them completely, though he could sometimes pronounce the same words correctly. Similarly, he would sometimes repeat the words correctly, but he would keep repeating them incessantly and mechanically until everyone around him was tired and bored.(...)

Opposition and even obedience lacked affection and comprehensibility. He was also remarkably insensitive to pain and did not ask for comfort and consolation when he was hurt.

Commentary on the clinical picture

Unlike previous distinguished commentators, to me the clinical picture does not seem clear at all. There is a global delay and there are relational and communicative difficulties; what strikes me is the child's oppositional and provocative behavior to the mother's demands and his "lack of interest in being understood". I think the situation will be clearer later.

Reorganized anamnestic information

Gravidance:no informations; Birth: no informations; Weight, condition at birth: no informations (but the sending doctor had excluded organic factors)

Feeding: *was particularly difficult from the very first days. The mother had tried with little success to breastfeed him for a few weeks until the baby almost died of starvation. It was necessary to use artificial milk. At the age of seven weeks he was found a nurse, but at that point he had no incentive to suck the breast, showed no desire to suck and continued in the same way. Afterwards he didn't want to take the milk from the bottle. When the solid food began, he refused to chew and absolutely refused anything that did not have the consistency of a soup; and he had to be forced to eat it anyway. After the second year there was an improvement in his desire to eat, which was a positive effect of the new nanny, but even so the difficulty persisted.*

Sleep: no information

Communication and Language: *The 'mechanical learning' of a number of new words after three years is reported. Mostly he just put together sounds in a meaningless way and repeated certain noises over and over again. When he spoke, he used his poor vocabulary incorrectly. But it wasn't only because of that he wasn't understandable: as I said before, he had no desire to be. He learned to walk in normal times. He was rather clumsy motorically. He didn't know how to use knives or scissors, but he knew how to use a spoon quite well when he ate.*

Sfinteric control: *there were difficulties with sphincter control. He acquired it much more easily with his new nanny, around the age of three, and at this point he was actually showing some 'ambition' and apprehension about it.*

Separation and stranger reaction: *Dick was ... indifferent to the presence or absence of his mother or nanny, but there is no information of any experience of separation.*

Emotional and affective aspects: *described as almost devoid of affectivity, emotional relationships with his environment and the ability to adapt to reality. From the earliest times he had shown signs of discomfort only rarely and to a low degree.*

Interest in people: *Despite the annotation that the good nanny had in some ways changed her development, the basic defects remained intact. With her and everyone else, Dick still did not establish friendly contact. So neither the nanny's tenderness nor her grandmother's was able to start a normal relationship. He was different from other children because of his lack of interest in his environment and the difficulty people had in getting in touch with his mind...*

Interest in objects: *The child had almost no interest, did not play, had no contact with his environment. He was indifferent to most of the objects and toys around him, he did not grasp their purpose or meaning. He had no special relationship with particular objects, as is usually seen even in the most inhibited children. (...) With one exception: he was interested in trains and stations, door handles and doors and in opening and closing them (...)*

Behavior: *Dick was oppositional to his mother, often doing just the opposite of what she expected of him. For example, if she could get him to repeat words, he would often cripple them completely, although he could sometimes pronounce the same words correctly. Similarly, he would sometimes repeat the words correctly, but he would keep repeating them incessantly and mechanically until everyone around him was tired and bored.(...)*

Environmental and caring aspects: *His mother felt a sense of coldness towards him from the beginning. At the end of the first year she was struck by the thought that the baby was not normal and this had an even worse effect on her disposition towards him. Moreover, since neither the father nor the (former) nanny had any tenderness towards him, Dick grew up in an environment unusually poor in love. At the age of two he had a new nanny who was good and loving and shortly afterwards he spent some time with his grandmother who was very loving towards him. These changes had a visible influence on his development.*

Other notes: *In his fourth year he was sensitive to reproaches. The nanny had found him masturbating and told him that it was bad and that he shouldn't do it. Also in this period Dick made some progress in adapting, mainly to external things and especially in mechanically learning a number of new words. He suffered from intestinal disorders, anus prolapsed and then hemorrhoids. Around five months and sometimes in the following periods, when he defecated or urinated, the baby showed a particular discomfort. The faeces were not hard, and the anus prolapsed and hemorrhoids did not seem to be enough to explain his anxiety, especially when urinating. Even during the sessions when he told me that he had to go to the bathroom he did so only after long hesitation and with great anxiety and had tears in his eyes.*

Comments on the anamnestic informations

We have no information about pregnancy, child-birth or birth conditions, except that the doctor had ruled out diseases or organic injuries. Nutrition was difficult, by the bottle after the failure of the mother's breast milk, we do not know for what possible reasons. Nutrition remained difficult for a long time, with refusal or inability to attach even to the nurse, after 7 weeks; afterwards he refused to chew solid food. We have no information about the physical condition at birth, about the stature-ponderal growth, but probably it will have been quite normal, since otherwise maybe there would have been a nod.

Towards the age of two there was an important environmental change, repeatedly stressed by Klein, due to the arrival of the new nanny and the involvement of the grandmother and the care of the child had an overall improvement, including also the alimentation. Thanks to the new nanny he also acquired sphincter control. Therefore, it seems that the child responded positively to the change, with a general recovery in development. The 'normal' age at which he took his first steps is not specified. The reported motor clumsiness could also suggest some motor immaturity.

The language seems to have appeared in the third year, after the environmental change. The news about the mother who made him repeat the words, with poor results, makes one think of suboptimal ways of communication and attention to the child, perhaps stressed by tests of abilities and performance requests, for the fear that it was not normal, manifested by the mother towards the year of age. Pre-verbal communication is not described. In addition to food and nutrition the rejection seems to have extended to people and objects, even with aspects frankly oppositional to the mother's demands, perhaps charged with apprehension and anxiety for fears that it was abnormal, as mentioned above.

The environmental characteristics do not seem negligible: until the arrival of the new nanny and grandmother the child seems to have lived in an emotional situation not good enough for his development, which seems to have even worsened in the second year of life.

There is no evidence of intestinal complications, whose influence on the baby's condition is minimized by Klein, although it is reported that after five months the emission of urine and faeces was linked to a particular anxiety of the baby that was also maintained afterwards.

The child therefore seems to have also had physical disturbances in addition to eating difficulties, particularly in the intestine and urinary tract, probably connected with painful experiences. Perhaps the rectal prolapse is not exactly painless and harmless and complicates the emission of feces by a lot, so much so as to justify perhaps the restlessness or even fear of the child when taking a poop.

Nothing is said about the events of attachment and separation and reaction to the stranger, but from the description of the first contact with Klein, a stranger, and the separation from the nanny who accompanied him, (see below: *The first time he came to me he showed no reaction to being left by the nanny*) it would seem that his feelings were as if they had been frozen, so to speak. But he began to show more normal reaction in the next sessions, as we'll see.

The first two years therefore seem to have been marked by negative and painful experiences in the face of which the environment did not seem to have had a helpful attitude towards the child, until the change that took place around the age of two, when a new nanny and grandmother took better care of him. This change, as we have seen, led to a certain general improvement and a recovery in development, which is stated by Klein herself.

There are enough elements to think of the first two years of life as characterized by predominantly negative experiences, in the face of which the child would seem to have reacted with an attitude of refusal towards food and then also towards the surrounding environment. It would seem possible to attribute a 'cumulative' traumatic effect to all these negative experiences lived by the child in the very first years of life. Even the improvement from the third year onwards following the environmental change appears compatible with post-traumatic pathogenesis.

In some aspects the situation described in this way recalls the experience of children adopted after a period of stay in an institution who resumed development after a developmental delay suffered in that period. (See Appendix 3 on so-called 'institutional autism')

The evolution during the six months of analysis

"The impression on the first visit was very particular. He left the nanny without any emotion and followed me into the room with complete indifference. Then he ran back and forth without purpose and also around me, several times, like around a piece of furniture, and showed no interest in any object in the room. The expression on his eyes and face was fixed, absent and without interest.(...) Dick's behaviour had no meaning or purpose and showed no sign of emotion or anxiety (...)

The first time he came to me, as I said above, he had no re-action to being left by the nanny. When I showed him the games I had prepared, he looked at them without the slightest interest. (...) (Of the two trains) he took the small one and ran it towards the window, saying 'Station'. (...) He left the train, ran into the space between the outer and inner door of the room, locked himself inside saying 'dark-ness' and then rushed back into the room. He repeated the scene several times. (...) Then he took the train again but soon came running back between the two doors. (...) He said 'nanny' twice. (M. Klein replied that she was coming). Dick repeats these words ("she's coming") almost correct-ly, even later.

The second time he behaved in the same way, but this time he ran out of the room into the dark entrance and brought the small train in and insisted on staying there and kept repeating "is Nanny coming?

In the third session he continued in the same way, except that, besides running in the entrance and between the doors, he also ran behind the chest of drawers. (...). He repeated the words Klein said, remembering them. For the first time he looked at the toys with interest (...) He said 'cut' and with the scissors he tried to cut black pieces out of a 'coal cart', but he didn't know how to use the scissors well. (Klein cut them for him) and he put the little pieces and the damaged wagon in a drawer, saying "go" (...) He ran between the two doors and scratched them a little bit with his nails (...) then ran away again, found the cupboard and threw himself inside.

At the beginning of the next session he cried, when the nanny left him (...), but he soon calmed down. This time he avoided the space between the doors, the walk-in closet and the corner and devoted himself to toys by examining them more closely and with evident initial curiosity. He found the wagon damaged the other time and the contents and pushed them away immediately, covering them with other things. (...) He took them out again and put them between the two doors. (...) Dick had discovered the sink and was very afraid of getting wet with water. With anxiety he dried his hand and mine, which he had immersed in the water, and immediately afterwards he showed the same anxiety while urinating. (...)

Once Dick took a man figurine and put it to his mouth saying "Tea daddy" (or "eat daddy"?) and then he wanted to drink.(...) He put the figurine in my hand and then everything back in the drawer(...) He saw some pieces of the freshly sharpened pencil left on my knees and said "Poor Mrs. Klein". And equally 'poor curtain', for the same reason (...)

For some time Dick avoided the walk-in cupboard and instead carefully examined the sink and the radiator, in every detail,(...) He then shifted his interest to new objects or things he had neglected for some time. He returned to the walk-in cupboard, now much more actively and with more curiosity and aggressiveness. He beat on it, scalped it and scratched it with a knife and sprayed water on it. He would examine the hinges of the door, the way it opened and closed, climb inside the wardrobe and ask for the names of the different parts, (...) remembering and using the words correctly.

In these months his attitude towards his mother and nanny became more normal and affectionate, he wanted to be with them and felt sorry when he was left. The relationship with his father also normalized, as it did with other people in general. Now he showed a desire to make himself understood, with his still struggling language that was increasing and his relationship with reality was stabilizing.

At this point, after six months of analysis,his development had resumed in all basic aspects, justifying a favorable prognosis.

Comment on the analysis period

It is therefore an astonishing development: in just six months of analysis the child, who had arrived seriously hampered in communication, relationship and social contact - so much so that he was retrospectively considered by many to be an autistic child - had a remarkable global change, with a resumption of development in all its aspects.

What could have happened? Klein has her explanations, but others will give others later (see below). For our part, we stress that going into analysis Dick suddenly finds himself in a situation in which a person dedicates himself to him for an hour, several times a week, observes him and pays attention to his behavior and what he does, talks to him about what he is doing, without asking him any particular questions or limits or rules, much less reproaches. The child is free to follow his initiatives with the objects and the environment at his disposal and to explore the situation. The novelty of all this is probably great compared to what the child is used to, and Dick (like many children in the first sessions of psychotherapy) seems to grasp it quickly and begins to explore the environment and things and the person who is with him, almost immediately establishing contact even verbal.

His first words, in the second session, refer to the nanny who accompanied him and left him there, thus touching on the theme of separation and of a stranger. In a rapid crescendo his words in the first sessions make explicit the desire for the nanny to come ("Tata is coming") until the arrival at the fourth session the child starts crying at the separation from the nanny, showing a normal and affective reaction to the separation, for a child who has not yet passed that phase. A delayed burst reaction that is not uncommon to see even in many nursery school children. He also began to use the material in the room and ask for the intervention of the person at his disposal.

We can think that the therapy situation (analytical situation) already had a particular 'therapeutic' effect, as well as the attention and contact on the part of Mrs Klein, although we are not obliged to believe that the child understood the meaning of her words (on the content of the interpretations see the comments of Lacan and Tustin in the last section). His behavior seems to have a meaning also using other levels of interpretation than those proposed by Klein, and it is conceivable that Dick certainly perceived the situation experienced as different from any other until then. The interest in him and the desire to get in touch with him by this adult person who was trying to understand children, their fears and their difficulties, seems to have touched him deeply.

We can think of it as a communication on an intuitive and non-verbal level that ran below the abstract level of words that however touched on very concrete and understandable things for the child, such as peeing, pooping, breaking things and fears. He could also enter into the various peripheries of the space at his disposal in order to experience them with an unthinkable freedom, out of there, almost in the manner of Maria Montessori and her discovery that children should be freed from the impediments placed by adults.

Progressively the child extended his exploration to the water, the bath and the use of it for his needs, always free to express himself and explore and always accompanied by that very special person who told him what he was thinking of and to whom he began to tell in a few words what came to his mind. They would share their experience and he would also take care of her, whether she got wet or dirty by being with him, and he would also show her the restorative cues that Klein elsewhere considers so important.

We can think that when the child arrived in therapy he was ready, thanks to the environmental change enjoyed with the new nanny and grandmother, to take advantage of the new experience that was proposed to him. In this way he was able, after a very short initial phase of mistrust, to get in touch with that lady and to progressively explore the relationship with her, with the objects and the space she made available to him. He thus had a global experience, of knowledge and containment, which until now had been wholly or partially prevented.

It is not surprising that in the following months the child showed clear signs of evolution and improvement even in the external environment, both in the communicative and linguistic as well as relational and behavioural fields. The experience with Klein had probably come at the right time and had accelerated an evolution that was already taking place and that probably also influenced the attitudes and climate in the child's family environment.

There is no news of the evolution of the child after those six months of analysis, as far as I know.

As for the language, from the very first sessions it does not really seem as compromised as it is described. Surely it is little used by the child but it seems to be acquired at the level of word-phrase and even two-word sentences, and also used to reflect and express thoughts and feelings.

In the sessions of the following months, interest in things, the environment, the names of things, all seems to grow rapidly in relation to the person who is now experienced as a companion of exploration. The child's previous rejection of contact seems to have loosened. The desire to communicate and to be understood that before seemed suffocated has emerged. The child seems to quickly recognize and use the opportunity of contact with a therapist who leaves him the possibility to explore the relationship with her as well.

The rapid and favorable evolution of the therapy more than to an 'autistic' child, as many have thought - and as would certainly now result by subjecting him to the tests used today - could make one think of a child with a developmental arrest reactive to environmental conditions.

Discussion about the diagnosis

At this point we can deal with the diagnosis which in Klein's words has various nuances: developmental delay, developmental inhibition, with a level of linguistic and intellectual development of about 15-18 months (compared to 4 years of age), Dementia praecox, schizophrenia. We are at the beginning of the 1930s, only a few years ago these diagnoses had been proposed and had spread in adult psychiatry and were beginning to be applied also in children, with diagnostic criteria that were used also for them, rather improperly.

The little 4-year-old Dick arrived with the diagnosis of dementia praecox (the oldest term for schizophrenia) but in the discussion of the case Klein disputes the absence of a regression, which is typical of these cases and instead emphasizes the presence of a developmental arrest. She excludes the presence of medical anomalies, also because of the positive evolution of the case with psychological treatment. But it also posits a diagnosis of psychosis, in particular schizophrenia, although with doubts and uncertainties, not having another existing psychiatric diagnosis available. Here Klein seems close to grasping the essential aspect (in my opinion) of the developmental problem but is influenced by the dominant ideas of adult psychiatry. The developmental problem will return many years later in DSM III at the point where it will establish, instead of the diagnosis of autism as a form of psychosis, the idea of a pervasive developmental disorder.

In hindsight, it is astonishing that in her discussion of the diagnosis Klein does not give value to the news about the environmental situation, which although in her description of the case she has carefully recorded and also attached some importance to them, it would seem. In her pathogenetic reconstruction, in fact, she only takes into account the 'internal' psychological vicissitudes of the child, based on her theories of development and internal psychological dynamics. She does not give any weight to the experiences lived by the child, even though she pointed out earlier as factors of delay and anomalies in his development. Even the hint that environmental modification, due to the arrival of the new nanny and grandmother, would have had a positive influence on development seems to be forgotten, due to the urgency of demonstrating her theories and the effect of her intervention. The case itself actually serves Klein to illustrate her theories, which in turn explain the child's behavior, in a closed circle that risks being vicious.

Also all his commentators seem to have given no importance to the news about the environmental context and the experiences lived by the child. The term she used regarding the emotional climate around the child, 'cold', anticipates the feedback from others, such as Kanner, which would have led to the ill-famed concept of 'refrigerator mother'. Opposite taboos, on both sides, led to a kind of anathema that has long prevented further studies of the family environment and its influence on development.

Case discussion

The reading of the case, in the way we have suggested, seems to give us the idea of an arrest, of a blockage of the child's development in the first months (as Klein had pointed out), to which at a certain point was also added a refusal and opposition to environmental demands. The development of the child, however, partially resumes after the second year of age, coinciding with the change in the way of care, and there is an emergence of language, perhaps in a less mechanical way than it seemed, and then the acquisition of sphincter control at the age of three, and also the flourishing of interest in some games, trains, handles and doors.

So the child is already in a recovery phase when he starts working with Klein. In the six months of analysis described, we are witnessing an acceleration of this recovery of development, which involves all levels, linguistic, symbolic, relational, affective. Probably it was the manifestation of something that was already underway and finds space to expand, for the rapid decrease in rejection and opposition, which were previously addressed to environmental demands. This seems to be the most visible aspect of the therapeutic experience. We would seem to be witnessing the liberation and the resumption of the child's evolutionary drive, which was first slowed down and arrested by the relational and affective environmental situation that was not favorable to the child's development.

It seems to have happened as in institutionalized children, where adoption and the start of a more normal living condition allows the resumption of development if the period in the institution has not been too long. So Dick was perhaps lucky enough to experience a positive environmental change in time to resume development and learning, first with his nanny and grandmother and then with Mrs. Klein. Otherwise perhaps his closure, rejection and withdrawal into a solipsistic world would have led to a stunting of mental development to a severe mental handicap.

Neither the diagnosis of dementia praecox, nor that of schizophrenia, nor that retrospectively postulated of autism (today they would say bureaucratically Autistic Spectrum Disorder) - with their heavy implications of an inborn, genetic causality - seem to me adequate to describe instead the vicissitudes of the development of little Dick in his environment. The described affectively negative conditions and the repeated (cumulative) traumatic experiences seem actually sufficient, as seen in institutionalized children, to explain the alterations and delays in his development.

The very rapid and positive response to the intervention does not seem compatible with a diagnosis of a serious genetic disease but rather with a developmental difficulty linked to the existence of initial environmental obstacles that were at least partially removed during the period of therapy and even before this allowing the recovery and overcoming of the blockage.

Thus it seems that the claim that it was a case of ante litteram autism is not perhaps as true as it seemed until now. Unless one thinks - as it is being thought from many quarters - that in reality the same diagnosis of autism, and even more so of the autistic spectrum, is in fact a diagnosis without validity, which has clouded the minds of many people and blocked the possibility of knowing more.

Note on Lacan and Tustin's comments

Both Klein's article and those of her commentators continue to receive rather high interest even in recent times. The Dick case was commented on by J Lacan, among others, in 'The Seminar' of 1954 [44], dedicated to technical aspects. Lacan appears impressed and admired by Klein's 'reckless and violent' use of interpretations. With these, according to him, she suddenly throws the child into the 'imaginary oedipal space', giving him access to the

---

[44]Jacques-Alain Miller *The Seminar of J.Lacan* Book 1: Freud's Papers on Technique 1953-1954

'symbolic register' that will activate the particularly positive evolution of the child. Discussing Klein's interpretations extensively, the French psychoanalyst even sets this case as a paradigmatic example of his tripartition of the psychic world in real/imaginary/symbolic.

Another famous psychotherapist, of English nationality, who wrote about the Dick case was F Tustin, in 1983 [45], who was particularly interested in diagnostic and interpretative aspects. Tustin seemed to be negatively affected by Klein's interpretations and felt the contents were wrong. She attributed the cause to a diagnostic error, that is, to having accepted, albeit with uncertainty and distinction, the diagnosis of schizophrenia with which the child had come to her. According to Tustin it was instead a typical case of Kanner's autism, which would have required interpretations of another type.

It is interesting that the child had a positive evolution despite the erroneous content, in the opinion of many, of the interpretations he received. Strangely enough, no one disputes or even examines Kanner's writing, which opens the door to the concept of autism, not only as a symptom but as a disease, and therefore to its diagnosis. The diagnosis of autism had imposed itself in all fields without finding the slightest resistance, if not Winnicott's comment quoted in another chapter of this book.

In psychoanalysis the content of the interpretations is often closely related to the analyst's theoretical refer-

---

[45]Tustin, F. (1983). Thoughts on autism with special reference to a paper by Melanie Klein. *Journal of Child Psychotherapy, 9*(2), 119–131. https://doi.org/10.1080/00754178308255043

ences, as Klein explicitly shows in the original writing of the work. Even Lacanian psychoanalysts who discuss Lacan's own comments on the case [46], say that today's interpretations would be different, for the different theoretical references of today. Often it is the banal 'hindsight', which allows many to feel superior to the men of the past.

But, as was once said, cases that go well are of little significance, perhaps because one is not sure what made them go well: much more so are cases that go wrong, failures, in which one can retrospectively recognize errors and learn from them.

All medicine, on the other hand, has gone and still goes on sometimes on the skin of patients, since it is known that medical errors and iatrogenic diseases, i.e. due to medical or health interventions, are not a marginal issue of current medicine. Autism is perhaps one of the biggest of these errors, even if this is stubbornly denied by almost all scientific and health authorities.

---

[46] M C LAZNIK, *Lacan e l'autismo,*Rivista di psicoanalisi, 2016, LXII, 3

Afterword I

Autistic bubbles

This book is not about autism, but about how to get rid of the deforming concept of autism and its derivatives such as the autism spectrum, to look instead at the phenomena that have been covered by this concept. How to take off the deforming lenses to look at the objects around us. I would say that for many years we have all been involved and possessed by this concept, so to speak, and inevitably deformed in our approach to people.

In the book I deal with the needs of young children and families with difficulties inherent in their psychic development, and I try to find ways to free the minds of parents and operators from something that prevents us from seeing these children as people, each with his or her own individuality, characteristics and experiences, to get in touch with them, to know them and to know their needs.

As suggested in the cover picture, what happens today is that the diagnosis seems to almost envelope the child in a semitransparent bubble that partially hides the child from sight. Parents, operators, teachers no longer see the child but the bubble that covers it, made of symptoms and characteristics and tables and comparisons with others. The parents themselves realize and regret that their attitude and their way of being with their child is no longer the same, but has been deeply altered by the diagnosis or their fears. The consequences for the child's relationship with those around him can be disastrous and accentuate his difficulties. Hence the need to burst those bubbles, to break the envelopes that imprison them.

I do not, however, deal in this book with older children and adults who grew up with this diagnosis, which was once used for much more serious situations on average than today, and I think I should somehow apologize and make up for it at least in part. Many have become adults with various degrees of social, relational, cognitive and linguistic disabilities, and therefore with a more or less serious handicap that prevents them from having an autonomous and independent life. This forces them to take advantage of the welfare services available, day and night centers, workshops. Their families now face not only the difficulties of everyday life but also the thought of "after us" in the not so distant future.

In addition to my young patients of the past, now grown up with ups and downs, who I have tried to help with my own strength, I have also taken care of older children and young adults over time. This happened in day centers or day group experiences, starting from a very first short experience at the ODA Day and Night Centre in Diacceto, Florence, during my residency. My first commitment was in the centre of Cerbaiola, near Empoli, many years ago, at the beginning of my activity. Then I was medical director of the AIABA centre in Florence in an intermediate period, and finally I followed the first initiatives of the 'Sipario' group, also in Florence, towards the end of my institutional activity.

Thinking back today, even in those situations, which mainly concerned young people with different psychic disabilities, the concept of autism does not seem to have been useful to assist them, if not to allow to have a higher operator/assisted ratio because the regional health institution gave a higher tuition for subjects diagnosed with autism. Actually the best results, in my opinion, both in individual therapies and in institutional situations, were those that came from taking care of people and their needs, being able to get in touch with them as persons independently from the diagnosis and theoretical knowledge about the characteristics deriving from the diagnosis. The important thing was the possibility to have different experiences in normal environments and with normal people, learning from living experience, and not from artificial and routine teachings.

The most evident and exciting demonstration for me was perhaps the experience with 'Sipario', today Social Cooperative 'I ragazzi di Sipario'[47], of which I witnessed the birth and the first years of evolution. In this experience, personally managed by some parents and operators, it was not the diagnosis that mattered but the possibility of involving the children in activities that put them in contact with the world and people in a new, interesting and non-routine

---

[47] I ragazzi di Sipario, Cooperativa Sociale https://prova.iragazzidisipario.it/

way. The important thing was the possibility to have different experiences in normal environments and with normal people, learning from living experience, and not from artificial and routine teachings. All the boys and girls, to my knowledge, felt very well with those experience, regardless of the diagnosis they had, which little by little lost importance and was finally forgotten.

The deep conviction that has matured in me is that the diagnosis in the field of neuropsychic development is secondary to the importance of recognition of the person and their individual personal characteristics, from the very first months until adulthood and at the end of life. In this regard, I am reminded of Adriano Milani Comparetti's teaching on the greater importance of prognosis compared to diagnosis, in the field of rehabilitation[48]. Without prejudice to the need to ensure medical diagnosis where possible and truly effective medical therapies.

The problems of psychic development and possible delays and disabilities do not depend so much on the diagnosis and characteristics of the illnesses as on the possibility of guaranteeing the subjects, regardless of the type and level of disability, have open and free experiences in contact with normal social environments where they can get to know the outside world and people. On this depends the fate of a possible development, which at first is often unpredictable.

---

[48] Milani Comparetti A, Gidoni EA., *Dalla parte del neonato: Proposte per una competenza prognostica.*Neuropsichiatria Infantile, fasc. 175. (1976)

Afterword II

Diagnosis and disability

At the end of this book I think I owe some explanations to the parents of the 'autistic' children who have grown up and become adults, who are perhaps puzzled by the possible change in the 'name' that has accompanied the life of their relative and theirs. Both to those whom I have personally followed in time and in the various contexts in which I found myself, and to those whom I have not known but are touched by my considerations and proposals. Many of their children have remained with different disabilities of various degrees in cognitive abilities, in their ability to adapt to different social situations, in language and communication skills. With some of them I have shared years of interventions and attempts to cure their difficulties and to favor the best possible evolution, with different outcomes and alternating vicissitudes.

Some parents, active in Associations that take care of their children's interests and try to promote useful initiatives for children like them, have reacted badly to the initiatives that I have started to change the approach to young children with developmental difficulties so far diagnosed as related to 'Autistic Spectrum Disorders'. As if they were afraid of the negative consequences of this change. It doesn't seem to me that there is this danger. Their children are now grown up, teenagers and adults, and their lives should not be affected by the change in diagnostic and care settings for young children, which seems necessary to me. The consequences of the change in care settings for children with developmental difficulties should not have a negative impact on older children and adults with neuro-psychological disabilities. Instead, they should help to have a more attentive approach to the individual needs of each person with disabilities. Attention to the group in such cases risks being detrimental to the individual, whose individuality is crushed by the group category.

Thinking back to my experience I can try to answer the question about the effect that a change in the conceptual and diagnostic approach can have on the understanding and assistance to the difficulties and disabilities of those persons who are now adolescents or adults and their families. The real problem is, in my opinion, that the diagnosis - as it is usually used now - at a certain point no longer serves to clarify and help to understand the difficulties of the individual person, but risks confusing him/her in the group of those who share the same diagnosis but maybe different needs. In this way problems, difficulties, needs, remedies are no longer focused on the individual but on the diagnostic category, on the group. Thus there is a tendency to explain behaviors, perhaps problematic and difficult to understand, attributing them to the diagnosed disease, thus losing the possibility of finding individual, contextual explanations. The attention to the diagnosis therefore risks crushing the needs of the individual. Bringing attention back to the individual can help to make him or her more visible and understandable, to free them from the constraints that unconsciously we often helped to create around them, wrapping them in what I have called the autistic bubble.

Moreover, the WHO's approach to identifying the best responses to the needs of people with disabilities is already based not so much on diagnosis as on the characteristics of disabilities. To this end, the International Classification of Functioning, Disability and Health (ICF) [49] has been defined, which is distinct from the Classification of Diseases (ICD), now in its eleventh version.

The changes of approach, even those proposed at international level, go on the road of putting the individual characteristics and needs of individuals before the characteristics of the carrier group of the same diagnostic category. It seems to me an acknowledgement that the individual has the right to have his or her specific needs known at that given moment, in that given environment, as an overall person, whereas now, with categorical diagnoses prevailing, is perhaps being put in the background. Prioritizing the category of diagnosys in itself tends to lead to all equal needs and equal responses, because it scotomizes and eliminates individual differences and needs (as is happening at

---

[49] OMS: International Classification of Functioning, Disability and Health, ICF (2001) - https://www.who.int/classifications/icf/en

the moment). Prioritizing the characteristics of the person tends to focus on needs that are never identical for the type of disability, but individualized according to the specific characteristics of the individual person in their specific environment. Similarly, different people, with or without disabilities and with different disabilities, may share needs arising from shared personal aspects and from a shared environmental situation.

Likewise, at the time, the need to change the psychiatric organization that was based on asylums and closed institutions was shared by all inmates regardless of their diagnosis and also by people without diagnosis, leading to the liberation of those locked up.

Losing the label of 'autistic' can therefore result not in damage, but in the advantage of having recognized the individual characteristics and needs, and individuals recognized as persons and not as bearers of diagnostic labels. All the more so if these are wrong.

REFERENCES

Autism Science Foundation, *Interviews-with dr Eric-London,* https://autismsciencefoundation.org/what-is-autism/autism-science/interviews-with-scientists/dr-eric-london-new-york-state-institute-for-basic-research-in-developmental-disabilities/

Benedetti G, *Sta per scoppiare la bolla dell'autismo?,* Toscana Medica, 8/2019

Benedetti G, *Appello a cambiare approccio ai bambini con difficoltà evolutive,* (Ago 2019) Change.org Petition http://chng.it/Zc6bChdLQj/

Bischi, Carini, Gardini, Tenti , *Sulle orme del caos,* Bruno Mondadori, (2004)

Burlingham, D., & Freud, A. (1944). Infants without families. Allen & Unwin.

Calia V., *autismo e disturbi dello spettro autistico.* Un pediatra per amico, 4/11/'19

Capozzi, F., *Autismo e la società 4.0: la psicoanalisi ha ancora diritto di parola?,* spiweb approfondimenti dossier, 12 ottobre 2017 https://www.spiweb.it/dossier/umani-robot-una-relazione-pericolosa-ottob.../

Czech H, *Hans Asperger, National Socialism, and "race hygiene" in Nazi-era Vienna, Molecular Autism*, 9,29 (2018)

Gillberg C., *The ESSENCE in child psychiatry: Early Symptomatic Syndromes Eliciting Neurodevelopmental Clinical Examinations,* Res Dev Disabil.Nov-Dec;31(6):1543-51 (2010)

Kanner L, *Child Psychiatry, 1957,* C C Thomas Publisher

Klein M.,*The Importance of Symbol-Formation in the Development of the Ego. Int. J. Psycho-Anal.*, 11:24-39 (1930)

Lasnik M.C., *Lacan e l'autismo* Rivista di Psicoanalisi, , LXII, 3 (2016)

Lombardo V., Meng-Chuan Lai & Baron-Cohen S, *Big data approaches to decomposing heterogeneity across the autism spectrum* ,Molecular Psychiatry, 24 , 1435-1450 (2019) https://www.nature.com/articles/s41380-018-0321-0/

London E., *Categorical diagnosis: a fatal flaw for autism research?,* Trends Neurosci. Dec;37(12):683-6 (2014)

London E.(interview by J Wright), *Alternative Diagnosis for Autism,* Spectrum, 2015, 1, https://www.spectrumnews.org/opinion/questions-for-eric-london-alternative-diagnoses-for-autism/

Luby J.L, *Editorial:The primacy of parenting,* J.Child Psychology and Psychiatry, 61,4 (2020)

Mecacci L, *Besprizornye,* Adelphi Edizioni, 2019

Meltzer, D., Bremner, J., Hoxter, S., Weddell, D. and Witten-berg, I. (1975). *Explorations in Autism: A Psycho-Analytical Study*, Karnac Books Ltd.

Milani Comparetti A, Gidoni EEA., *Dalla parte del neona-to: Proposte per una competenza prognostica.* Neurop-sichiatria Infantile, fasc. 175. (1976)

Montessori M, *The Discovery of the Child* (1948) Madras, Kalakshetra,

Miller J A *The Seminar of J.Lacan* Book 1: Freud's Papers on Technique 1953-1954

Muller R A, Amaral DG., *Editorial: Time to give up on Au-tism Spectrum Disorder?*, Autism Res. Jan;10(1):10-14, (2017)

Reichow B., Hume K, Barton EE., Boyd BA., *Early inten-sive behavioral intervention (EIBI) for young children with autism spectrum disorders (ASD)*. Cochrane Data-base of Systematic Reviews 2018, Issue 5. Art. No.: CD009260. DOI: 10.1002/14651858.CD009260.pub3

Rutter M, e al.,*Longitudinal Studies Using a "Natural Ex-periment" Design: The Case of Adoptees From Roma-nian Institutions* Journal of the American Academy of Child & Adolescent Psychiatry51,8,762-770 (2012)

Sipario (I ragazzi di) Cooperativa Sociale, https://prova.iragazzidisipario.it/

Sheffer E., *Asperger's Children: The Origins of Autism in Nazi Vienna* - New York: W.W. Norton & Company, (2018)

Society for Chaos Theory, *Nonlinear Dynamics in Psy-chology and Life Science,* http://www.societyforchaostheory.org/home/

Spitz R., (1958). The *first year* of life: A psychoanalytic study of normal and deviant development of object relations. New York: International Universities.

Szasz, T., *The Myth of Mental Illness,* Harper & Row New York 1961

SINPIA (Società Italiana Neuropsichiatria Infanzia Adolescenza), *Linee guida sull'autismo*, 2011, Erikson Ed.

Tribulato E., *Autismo e gioco libero autogestito,* Franco Angeli editore,(2013)

Tustin F., (1983) Thoughts on autism with special reference to a paper by Melanie Klein. *Journal of Child Psychotherapy, 9*(2), 119–131.
https://doi.org/10.1080/00754178308255043

Vigotsky L S, (1934), *Thought and Language*, The MIT Presse

Waterhouse L., *Rethinking Autism,* Academic Press, 2012

Waterhouse L., Gillberg C., *Why Autism Must be Taken Apart*Autism Dev Disord. ul;44(7):1788-92, (2014)

Waterhouse L, London E, Gillberg C, *The ASD diagnosis has blocked the discovery of valid biological variation in neurodevelopmental social impairment*Autism Research Volume 10, Issue 7 (2017)

Waterhouse L, London E & Gillberg C, *Autism Spectrum Disorder Validity,* Review Journal of Autism and Developmental Disorders, Volume 3, Issue 4, pp 302–329 (2016)

WHO: International Classification of Functioning, Disability and Health, ICF (2001) -
https://www.who.int/classifications/icf/en

Winnicott D., cit da Brutti, Scotti, *Editoriale,* Quaderni di
  Psicoterapia infantile, n3, pag12 - 1980
Zappella, M *Difficoltà diagnostiche in bambini con distur-
  bi del neurosviluppo* Autismo e Disturbi dello Svilup-
  po',17(2):169-183 (2019)
Zeanah C. H., Sonuga-Barke E.J.S. *Editorial: The effects of
  early trauma and deprivation on human development –
  from measuring cumulative risk to characterizing spe-
  cific mechanisms,* J.Child Psychol Psychiatry.   2016
  Oct;57(10):1099-102. doi: 10.1111/jcpp.12642.
Zeanah C H., Humphreys K. L, *Child Abuse and Neclect*,
  JAACAP 2018,57,9,637

Acknowledgements

I am grateful to my wife Paola Baragatti, an artist in Florence, and my sister Maria Donata Benedetti, a neurologist in Verona, for having read the manuscript and suggested important corrections. Dr. Sara Francesconi from Pistoia has provided valuable support: without her stimulus the book would not have been born.

I have to thank my wife, my sons Saverio, Martino, Emiliano, and my daughter Simona, for having endured, over the years, the setbacks of my professional life.

My friend Scott Wing, an architect from San Francisco, CA, gave me precious help reading and correcting online the English version.